Anaesthesia

Commissioning Editor: Michael Parkinson
Development Editor: Clive Hewat
Project Manager: Elouise Ball
Design Direction: Erik Bigland
Illustrator: Joanna Cameron
Illustration Buyer: Merlyn Harvey

Anaesthesia

Michael Nathanson MRCP FRCA
Consultant Anaesthetist, Queen's Medical
Centre, Nottingham, UK

Ravi Mahajan DM FRCA
Professor and Honorary Consultant, Anaesthesia
and Critical Care, City Hospital, Nottingham, UK

With Contributions by

Bernard Riley MBE BSc FRCA
Consultant in Adult Critical Care, Queen's
Medical Centre, Nottingham, UK

Jo Lamb FRCA
Consultant Anaesthetist, Queen's Medical
Centre, Nottingham, UK

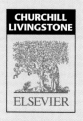

CHURCHILL
LIVINGSTONE

ELSEVIER

EDINBURGH LONDON NEW YORK OXFORD PHILADELPHIA
ST LOUIS SYDNEY TORONTO 2006

CHURCHILL LIVINGSTONE
ELSEVIER

1004 994 120

© 2006 Elsevier Limited. All rights reserved.

The right of Michael Nathanson and Ravi Mahajan to be identified as authors of this work has been asserted by them in accordance with the Copyright, Designs and Patents Act 1988

ISBN 10: 0443070261
ISBN 13: 9780443070266

British Library Cataloguing in Publication Data
A catalogue record for this book is available from the British Library

Library of Congress Cataloging in Publication Data
A catalog record for this book is available from the Library of Congress

Note
Knowledge and best practice in this field are constantly changing. As new research and experience broaden our knowledge, changes in practice, treatment and drug therapy may become necessary or appropriate. Readers are advised to check the most current information provided (i) on procedures featured or (ii) by the manufacturer of each product to be administered, to verify the recommended dose or formula, the method and duration of administration, and contraindications. It is the responsibility of the practitioner, relying on their own experience and knowledge of the patient, to make diagnoses, to determine dosages and the best treatment for each individual patient, and to take all appropriate safety precautions. To the fullest extent of the law, neither the Publisher nor the Authors assumes any liability for any injury and/or damage to persons or property arising out or related to any use of the material contained in this book.
The Publisher

ELSEVIER
your source for books, journals and multimedia in the health sciences
www.elsevierhealth.com

Working together to grow libraries in developing countries

www.elsevier.com | www.bookaid.org | www.sabre.org

ELSEVIER   **BOOK AID International**   **Sabre Foundation**

The Publisher's policy is to use **paper manufactured from sustainable forests**

PREFACE

The practice of anaesthesia encompasses many physiological principles, applied pharmacology, practical techniques, knowledge of equipment and physics, general (internal) medicine – and requires a working knowledge of surgical procedures. The fact that modern anaesthesia looks, to other medical practitioners, like a simple process and nearly always routine, is due to the complex amalgam of skills and abilities that anaesthetists learn during their whole career but particularly during their early training.

It is often stated that anaesthesia was first performed in 1846 in Boston, USA. In fact the state of anaesthesia was almost certainly induced some years before this. However, the public demonstration of ether anaesthesia in October 1846 was rapidly followed by the use of first ether and then chloroform in other countries. The use of local anaesthetics began a few years later. The revolution in surgery and the improvement in the humanity of care cannot be overstated. Many of the principles that guided the first practitioners still apply today. The development of new drugs and techniques has not changed the basic (patho)physiological state of general anaesthesia. (Indeed, our knowledge of the mechanism of general anaesthesia is still incomplete.) However, the number of techniques and drugs leaves many newcomers bewildered.

We hope that the new trainee in anaesthesia will use this book as a primer in anaesthesia. It is intended as an introduction to the speciality. The learning curve at the beginning of anaesthetic training is steep and many books are available to guide the more experienced trainee during their search for knowledge. We have tried to produce a pocket book that new trainees can carry around with them in their coat pockets when they visit patients on the wards, in the pre-assessment clinic or in recovery, HDU or ICU and in their greens, bags or briefcases when they are in theatre. As well as providing an introduction to the relevant physiology, drugs, equipment and techniques, we have included a number of action plans to help trainees in times of apparent crisis. This book does not provide details on anaesthesia for more complex, specialized surgery such as cardiac surgery and neurosurgery. Nor does it cover anaesthesia for obstetrics or chronic pain management. Care of children is also not covered, although many of the principles are, of course, the same.

We are indebted to our colleagues Dr Jo Lamb and Dr Bernard Riley for their contributions. Dr Riley has written the chapter on Intensive Care Medicine that, like the rest of this book, acts as an introduction to this topic. Intensive Care Medicine is correctly a speciality in its own right. However, new anaesthetists need to be aware of the function of the ICU and HDU. Dr Lamb has provided readers with an introduction to anaesthesia training so that newcomers may know what will happen to them and what will be expected of them as they progress through the early stages of their careers.

Most anaesthetists arrive at the speciality after some experience in another medical field. Suddenly being confronted with a completely new subject about which they have little experience or knowledge makes many newcomers uncomfortable. The speed with which most new trainees pick up the essential elements of safe anaesthesia is predominantly due to the excellent training they receive during their first SHO attachment. No book can replace the educational opportunities of 'on-the-job' learning. We hope you will find this book useful in augmenting the knowledge and skills you learn during your first few weeks and months.

CONTENTS

BASIC SCIENCE

PHYSIOLOGY

CARDIOVASCULAR PHYSIOLOGY

Knowledge of the cardiovascular system along with the respiratory system is essential both to providing safe anaesthesia and to understanding the many changes which take place in these systems during general, regional and local anaesthesia.

SYSTEMIC AND PULMONARY CIRCULATIONS

The systemic and pulmonary circulations form a double loop. Table 1.1 shows the pressures and haemoglobin oxygen saturation of the blood in the different chambers of the heart and the large vessels in the normal (healthy) state.

CONDUCTION SYSTEM OF THE HEART

The electrical impulse originates from spontaneous discharge of cells in the sino-atrial (SA) node which is situated at the junction of right atrium and superior vena cava. The SA node discharges at a rate of 70–80 bpm. The impulse travels through the right atrium to the atrio-ventricular (AV) node, and then into the bundle of His, which divides into right and left bundle branches. These divide into a network of conducting fibres (Purkinje fibres) that spread throughout the ventricular musculature. The cells in the SA node assume the role of cardiac pacemaker due to their faster intrinsic rate of discharge compared with cells in the rest of the heart. The pacemaker cells contain ion channels (calcium, sodium and potassium) and adrenoreceptors (β). The automaticity or the rate of spontaneous depolarization of the pacemaker cells is influenced by:

- sympathetic activity
- parasympathetic activity
- temperature
- oxygenation
- potassium concentration
- other electrolyte imbalances
- pathological processes.

Sympathetic fibres innervate the atria, the ventricles and all of the conducting system. Their actions are mediated predominantly by β_1 adrenoreceptors. The parasympathetic fibres (from the vagus nerve) innervate predominantly the SA node and atria. Stimulation of the vagus nerves slows SA node discharge (bradycardia) and stimulation of sympathetic nervous system increases SA node discharge (tachycardia). Overall the inhibitory parasympathetic system predominates.

TABLE 1.1 Pressure and haemoglobin oxygen saturation in great vessels and chambers of the heart

	Pressure (mmHg)	Oxygen saturation (%)
Inferior vena cava	0–8 (mean)	75–80
Superior vena cava	0–8 (mean)	65–75
Right atrium	0–8 (mean)	70–80
Right ventricle	20–30/0–8 (sys/dia)	70–80
Pulmonary artery	20–30/4–12 (sys/dia)	70–80
Left atrium	5–12 (mean)	94–100
Left ventricle	100–140/4–12 (sys/dia)	94–100
Aorta	100–140/60–90 (sys/dia)	94–100

CARDIAC OUTPUT

Cardiac output (CO) is the amount of blood leaving the heart per minute.

$$CO = \text{heart rate} \times \text{stroke volume}$$

The stroke volume is determined by:

- preload
- myocardial contractility
- afterload.

The ventricular function curve or Starling curve (see Figure 1.1) describes the relationship between the length of the cardiac muscle fibres at the end of diastole and the force of contraction. The greater the length of the muscle (that is – the degree of stretch of the cardiac muscle at the end of diastole) the greater the contractile tension it develops. An increase in venous return (or preload) stretches the muscle fibres, increasing their contractility and increasing the cardiac output. Afterload is determined by the systemic vascular resistance (SVR). The relationship between cardiac output, mean arterial pressure (MAP), central venous pressure (CVP) and SVR is:

$$CO = (MAP–CVP)/SVR$$

Atrial contraction contributes 20–30% of ventricular filling, the rest occurs passively. The atrial component is lost during atrial fibrillation leading to reduced ventricular filling and reduced stroke volume. Other factors which reduce ventricular filling are:

- increased heart rate (reduced diastolic time)
- mitral stenosis
- ischaemic heart disease
- hypertrophic cardiomyopathies.

During systole, left ventricular contraction creates a stroke volume of ~70 ml. The ratio of stroke volume to end-diastolic volume is called the ejection fraction, and can be estimated non-invasively using echocardiography. An ejection fraction of less than 0.4 indicates a significant abnormality of left ventricular function.

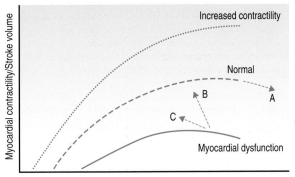

Fig. 1.1 Starling curve. Normally myocardial force of contraction increases with increase in ventricular filling pressure. Overstretching of the fibres (overload) decreases the contractility (A). The curve is flattened and shifted to the right in myocardial dysfunction, and it is steeper and shifted to the left during increased contractility (sympathetic stimulation). Use of inotropes in failing myocardium attempts to shift the curve towards normal (B), and use of vasodilators (C) may improve contractility by reducing the filling pressure and the afterload.

Preload

The systemic veins are the capacitance vessels of the body. About 60% of the total blood volume is contained in small veins and venules. The compliance of the venous system is regulated by vascular tone controlled by the autonomic nervous system. Constriction of the veins due to increased sympathetic activity can have the same effect as adding 1 litre of blood to the circulation. With dilatation the veins can accommodate up to 75% of the total blood volume. Factors decreasing preload (venous return) are:

- hypovolaemia
- haemorrhage
- autonomic neuropathy
- central neuraxis anaesthesia
- general anaesthesia
- positive pressure ventilation of the lungs.

During positive pressure ventilation, hypovolaemia and changes in posture, compensatory mechanisms tend to increase the tone of the veins leading to an increase in venous return. These mechanisms are impaired during spinal and epidural anaesthesia, in patients with autonomic neuropathy or in patients receiving vasodilatory drugs. General anaesthesia also reduces the capacity to compensate for changes in central venous volume. Because of these factors, patients undergoing anaesthesia are more likely to develop decreased cardiac output and hypotension in response to hypovolaemia, haemorrhage or changes in posture.

Afterload
The factors that decrease afterload (systemic vascular resistance) are:

- anaemia
- exercise
- hyperthyroidism
- arterio-venous shunts
- vasodilators.

The factors that increase the afterload are:

- polycythaemia
- hypothermia
- vasoconstriction
- application of tourniquets
- sympathetic stimulation.

Contractility
Factors that can affect myocardial contractility are given in Table 1.2.

MYOCARDIAL METABOLISM AND BLOOD SUPPLY

A balance must exist between oxygen consumption and oxygen supply to prevent myocardial ischaemia. The oxygen consumption of the myocardial cells is increased by extra work due to an increased heart rate, increased force of contractility or increased ventricular wall tension (end diastolic pressure).

TABLE 1.2 Factors that change myocardial contractility

Factors that increase myocardial contractility

Increased preload
Decreased afterload
Sympathetic stimulation
Inotropes:
– β_1 agonists
– phosphodiesterase inhibitors
– glucagon
– calcium

Factors that decrease myocardial contractility

Decreased preload
β blockade
Calcium channel blockade
Electrolyte imbalance
Myocardial ischaemia
Uraemia
Sepsis
Cardiomyopathy
Metabolic acidosis

Myocardial oxygen supply is determined by:

- aortic diastolic pressure
- left ventricular end diastolic pressure
- coronary artery calibre
- arterial oxygen content
- heart rate (increased heart rate decreases oxygen supply).

Coronary circulation

Approximately 4–5% of the total cardiac output (about 200–250 ml/min) of blood is supplied to the myocardium through the coronary circulation. The major coronary arteries are epicardial vessels which have a large diameter and low resistance. These supply the high resistance intramyocardial vessels. The majority of the blood supply to the myocardium occurs during diastole because the intramyocardial pressure is lowest at this time. The duration of diastole, which shortens during a tachycardia, determines coronary blood flow.

DISTRIBUTION OF CARDIAC OUTPUT

Blood leaving the heart is distributed to the various organs (see Table 1.3).

BLOOD PRESSURE

Blood pressure is determined by the cardiac output and systemic vascular resistance.

$$MAP = CO \times SVR$$

A number of regulatory mechanisms control blood pressure.

Rapidly acting mechanisms

The reflexes important in rapid adjustment of blood pressure are:

- Baroreceptor reflexes, in particular during changes in posture; blunted by volatile anaesthetics.
- Atrial reflexes, causing vasodilatation and tachycardia.
- Central nervous system ischaemic reflex or Cushing reflex, activated during ischaemia of the central vasomotor centre; leads to intense sympathetic nervous system activity.

TABLE 1.3 Distribution of the cardiac output at rest

Organ	Cardiac output
Brain	12%
Heart	4%
Liver	24%
Kidneys	20%
Skeletal muscle	23%
Skin	6%
Intestines	8%

Intermediate response mechanisms

Hormonal mechanisms to provide moderately rapid control of the blood pressure:

- Catecholamines – norepinephrine, (α-agonist), constricts arteries and veins independent of their neural supply; epinephrine, (β-agonist), increases myocardial contractility.
- Renin-angiotensin system – renin, released from the kidneys as a result of a reduction in renal perfusion initiates the formation of angiotensin I, converted to angiotensin II in the lungs (angiotensin converting enzyme), a vasoconstrictor and stimulates the secretion of aldosterone, conserves sodium and retains water.
- Atrial natriuretic peptide – stored in atrial myocytes, released in response to increased vascular volume (atrial distension); decreases blood pressure by peripheral dilatation, natriuresis and diuresis.

Long-term mechanisms

Changes in sodium and water excretion by the kidneys and the long-term effects of the renin-angiotensin system.

PULMONARY CIRCULATION

The pulmonary circulation is a low-pressure, high-flow system. Its principle functions are:

- transport of blood through the lungs for gas exchange
- drug metabolism
- removal of norepinephrine and prostaglandins
- inactivation of acetylcholine and bradykinin
- reservoir for the left ventricle
- filtration of venous drainage.

A hypoxic gas mixture in the alveoli causes pulmonary vasoconstriction (hypoxic pulmonary vasoconstriction). This is a protective response that diverts the blood from less ventilated (atelectatic) areas to the ventilated ones, thus minimizing the V/Q mismatch. Inhaled anaesthetic agents and some vasodilators inhibit this response and can increase V/Q mismatch.

RESPIRATORY PHYSIOLOGY

Four aspects of lung physiology have major implications in anaesthesia:

- mechanics of ventilation
- control of breathing
- lung volumes
- pulmonary gas exchange.

MECHANICS OF VENTILATION

The main muscle of breathing is the diaphragm, which is responsible for 75% of air movement during normal tidal breathing. It is innervated by the phrenic nerve (C3, C4, C5). During quiet breathing, the intercostal muscles remain largely inactive; however, during laboured breathing or dyspnoea, the intercostals as well as the accessory muscles of breathing become active. The abdominal muscles become active during forced exhalation for certain manoeuvres such as coughing.

Work of breathing

In terms of oxygen, the cost of breathing at rest is less than 5% of the total oxygen consumed by the body. In respiratory failure, the cost of breathing can increase to up to 25%. The work of breathing is required to overcome the elastic recoil of lungs (as assessed by compliance) and the resistance to flow (airway resistance).

Compliance is the change in volume per unit change in pressure. The normal compliance of the lungs and chest wall is $0.1 \text{ L/cmH}_2\text{O}$. The tendency of the lungs to collapse is opposed by a thin lining of surfactant which reduces surface tension. Factors that affect compliance are those which affect the thoracic cage, the alveolar wall, or the surfactant.

The resistance of the airways depends on their length and calibre. The presence of a tracheal tube adds to the resistance. This can be an important factor in children. The flow of air in the respiratory airways is either laminar (streamlined) or turbulent. Turbulence in air flow adds to the airway 'resistance'. Factors affecting resistance are those which affect the patency of the airway lumen (presence of tumours, foreign body, debris, blood or secretions) or those which affect the calibre of bronchioles including drugs which cause bronchoconstriction or bronchodilatation.

CONTROL OF BREATHING

The control of ventilation is a complex phenomenon which requires the integration of many parts of the central and peripheral nervous systems. The medulla oblongata in the brainstem contains inspiratory and expiratory centres which respond to central and peripheral chemoreceptors. The reticular activating system in the mid-brain and cerebral cortex affect the pattern of breathing and certain reflexes, such as swallowing, coughing and vomiting, directly influence ventilation.

Chemical control of ventilation

Alveolar ventilation is adjusted to maintain optimal PaO_2, $PaCO_2$ and H^+ ion concentrations. The $PaCO_2$ is a major factor in regulation of ventilation. Approximately 80% of the ventilatory response to inhaled carbon dioxide is influenced by central chemoreceptors, located in medulla. They respond to changes in H^+ ion concentration, which do not readily cross the blood–brain barrier. Carbon dioxide does cross the blood–brain barrier, however, and diffuses into the CSF to form H^+ ions in presence of carbonic anhydrase. These ions stimulate the central chemoreceptors to increase ventilation. After 3–6 h, the stimulant effect of carbon dioxide on ventilation is neutralized by active transport of bicarbonate ions into the CSF from blood to bring the CSF pH back to a normal value.

The peripheral chemoreceptors are located in the carotid and aortic bodies. They respond to changes in PaO_2, $PaCO_2$ and H^+ ion concentration. It is the PaO_2 (the partial pressure of oxygen in blood)

TABLE 1.4 Ventilatory response to carbon dioxide

Increased response
Hypoxia
Metabolic acidosis
Salicylate poisoning
Anxiety
Cirrhosis

Decreased response
Metabolic alkalosis
Sleep
Denervation of peripheral chemoreceptors
Opioid agonists
Volatile anaesthetic agents

and not the oxygen saturation that determines the stimulation of peripheral chemoreceptors. A PaO_2 below 8 kPa stimulates ventilation.

It is mainly the central, but also the peripheral chemoreceptors, that contribute to increased ventilation during carbon dioxide inhalation. The factors which can affect ventilatory response to carbon dioxide are given in Table 1.4.

LUNG VOLUMES

Tidal volume and minute volume

The tidal volume (V_T) is the amount of air that is inhaled and then exhaled during each respiratory cycle. During normal, quiet respiration it ranges between 10–15 ml/kg bodyweight (450–750 ml in adults). The tidal volume and respiratory rate (RR) determine the minute volume.

$$\text{Minute volume} = V_T \times RR$$

Sedatives, opioids and anaesthetics tend to reduce the tidal volume and respiratory rate and therefore the minute ventilation. An increase in minute ventilation during spontaneous breathing during anaesthesia can be due to oxygen lack, carbon dioxide excess, irritation of the respiratory tract or a reflex response to surgical stimulation.

Dead space

The respiratory passages extend from the nostrils and mouth down to the respiratory bronchioles and comprise the anatomical dead space. The normal value for the anatomical deadspace in adults is 150–200 ml. The alveolar deadspace is that part of the alveolar airspace which is ventilated but does not come into close enough

TABLE 1.5 Factors affecting dead space

Increased dead space
Old age
Upright position
Increased respiratory rate
Bronchodilators
Lung disease
Haemorrhage
Pulmonary embolism
IPPV
Chronic obstructive airway disease
Anaesthetic circuits and apparatus

Decreased dead space
Tracheostomy

proximity to blood in the pulmonary capillaries to contribute to gas exchange. The physiological dead space is the fraction of the tidal volume not used for gaseous exchange and is the combination of the anatomical and alveolar deadspaces. The factors affecting physiological dead space are given in Table 1.5.

Alveolar ventilation
This is the part of the tidal volume which takes part in gas exchange.

Alveolar ventilation = $(V_T - \text{physiological dead space}) \times RR$

Alveolar ventilation is invariably reduced by anaesthesia with spontaneous ventilation and this leads to arterial hypoxaemia as well as carbon dioxide retention. It is usual, therefore, to administer an inspired oxygen concentration of at least 33% in all anaesthetic gas mixtures.

Vital capacity
The vital capacity is the volume of air that can be exhaled maximally after a maximal inspiration. It includes the tidal volume, the inspiratory reserve volume (the amount of air that can be further inspired after normal inspiration), and the expiratory reserve volume (the amount of air that can be further exhaled after normal expiration). In a healthy adult the vital capacity ranges from 3–4.5 litres. A normal vital capacity is important for coughing and airway clearance. Factors that can reduce vital capacity are given in Table 1.6.

The ratio of the forced expiratory volume in one second (FEV_1) to the forced vital capacity (FVC) is about 0.75 in a healthy adult. A reduction in this ratio signifies obstructive airway disease. An

---

TABLE 1.6 Factors reducing vital capacity

Old age
Supine position
Reduced muscle power – myopathies, myasthenia gravis, residual effect of neuromuscular blockers, nerve palsies
Chronic airways obstruction
Abdominal distension and splinting of the diaphragm – ascitis, bowel obstruction, bowel perforation, abdominal pain
Following thoracic or abdominal surgery

FEV_1 of less than 1 L signifies severe respiratory disease with implications during anaesthesia and in the postoperative period.

Functional residual capacity

The functional residual capacity (FRC) is the volume of gas held in the lungs at the end of a normal expiration. It includes the expiratory reserve volume and the residual volume (the volume of air that remains in the lungs after a maximal expiratory effort). The normal FRC is 2.5–3.5 L. With pre-oxygenation, oxygen in the FRC can provide a reservoir that can be taken up by the blood during apnoea.

Closing capacity

Closing capacity is the volume of the lungs at which airways begin to close during expiration. Its value is lowest in the late teens and above this age it progressively increases. If the FRC is less than the closing capacity some airways will always be closed during normal tidal breathing. Blood will pass (or shunt) through the closed (non-ventilated) areas of the lung and arterial PO_2 will fall. In subjects with normal lungs, closing capacity becomes equal to FRC in the sixties (and in the forties when supine). Factors which increase closing capacity (Table 1.7) and/or decrease FRC (Table 1.8) cause arterial hypoxaemia.

TABLE 1.7 Factors increasing closing capacity (promote airway closure)

Smoking and COPD
Obesity
Abdominal distension
Rapid intravenous transfusion
Left ventricular failure
Recent surgery

TABLE 1.8 Factors reducing functional residual capacity

Supine position
Loss of muscle tone
Anaesthesia
Abdominal distension
Restrictive lung disease
Pulmonary fibrosis
Left ventricular failure
Abdominal pain
Adult respiratory distress syndrome

PULMONARY GAS EXCHANGE

Gas is exchanged in the lungs by passive diffusion across the alveolar-capillary membrane. This consists of the alveoli, interstitial fluid and the capillary endothelium. The normal mixed venous (pulmonary artery) partial pressure of oxygen is around 5.3 kPa while the alveolar PO_2 is around 14 kPa. Therefore oxygen diffuses along a gradient of 8–9 kPa. The normal mixed venous partial pressure of carbon dioxide is 6.1 kPa and the alveolar PCO_2 is 5.3 kPa, giving a gradient of 0.8 kPa for carbon dioxide diffusion. However, carbon dioxide diffuses 20 times more rapidly than oxygen. Thickening of the alveolar capillary membrane, for example by pulmonary fibrosis or from left ventricular failure, impairs the diffusion of gases.

Relationship between ventilation and perfusion

Both ventilation and perfusion of the lungs are better at the bases, but the gradient up the lungs is greater for perfusion, so that there is almost no perfusion of the apices in the upright position but the apices are ventilated to some extent. The normal alveolar ventilation (V) in an adult is 4 L/min and total perfusion (Q) about 5 L/min. This gives a ventilation/perfusion ratio (V/Q) for the whole lung of 4/5 = 0.8. The relative differences in ventilation and perfusion at the top and bottom of the lung produce regional variations in the V/Q ratios. With blood flow being negligible at the apex of the lung the V/Q ratio here is around 3.6, and at the bases where the ventilation is exceeded by blood flow, the V/Q ratio is around 0.63. Alveoli with a high (>1) V/Q ratio contribute to the alveolar dead space, whilst those with low (<1) V/Q ratio add to the shunt. The causes for V/Q mismatch are given in Table 1.9.

A shunt of 1–2% of cardiac output occurs at rest, but this may increase to 5–10% during anaesthesia.

TABLE 1.9 Factors affecting the V/Q ratio

Increased V/Q ratio (increased dead space)

IPPV
Increased minute ventilation
Hypotension
Low cardiac output
Pulmonary embolism

Decreased V/Q ratio (increased shunt)

Reduced minute ventilation
Atelectasis and lung collapse
Small tidal volumes
Pulmonary infection
Contused, damaged or oedematous lungs

TRANSPORT OF GASES IN THE BLOOD

Oxygen

A small proportion of the total oxygen carried in the blood is
dissolved in the plasma ($0.3\,ml/100\,ml$ of blood at PaO_2 of
$13.3\,kPa$). The majority of the oxygen is carried combined with
haemoglobin. Approximately $1.34\,ml$ of oxygen is carried by $1\,g$ of
fully oxygenated haemoglobin and at an arterial PaO_2 of $13.3\,kPa$,
haemoglobin is 97.5% saturated.

$$\text{Oxygen content} = \text{Hb} \times SaO_2/100 \times 1.34\,ml/100\,ml \text{ blood}$$

Thus, $15\,g$ of haemoglobin present in $100\,ml$ of blood can carry
approximately $19.5\,ml$ of oxygen. The oxygen flux is the amount of
oxygen leaving the left ventricle per minute.

$$\text{Oxygen flux} = \text{oxygen content} \times \text{cardiac output}$$

With a cardiac output at rest of $5\,L/min$, approximately 1
litre of oxygen leaves the left ventricle per minute. The oxygen
requirement of the body is about $250\,ml/min$ and the remaining oxygen returns to the lungs in the mixed venous blood (75%
saturated).

Oxygen dissociation curve

The relationship between the partial pressure of oxygen in
blood and percent saturation of haemoglobin with oxygen is
described by the oxygen–haemoglobin dissociation curve
(Figure 1.2). At the upper flat part of the curve changes in
PO_2 have relatively little effect on the oxygen saturation of the
haemoglobin, and, therefore, on the blood oxygen content. Over
the lower, more vertical part of the curve, changes in PO_2 have a

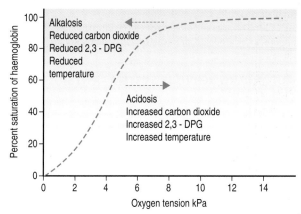

Fig. 1.2 The shape of the oxyhaemoglobin dissociation curve is sigmoid. This promotes uptake of oxygen in the lungs and its download at the tissue levels. While the flatter upper portion allows significant reduction in oxygen tension without much effect on oxygen saturation, at the steeper portion of the curve a small decrease in oxygen tension can cause large decreases in oxygen saturation. The factors that cause leftward shift (increased affinity of haemoglobin for oxygen) or rightward shift (decreased affinity) of this curve are shown.

marked effect on the oxygen saturation. The steep portion of the oxygen–haemoglobin curve allows small changes in the PaO_2 to result in the transfer of large amounts of oxygen from haemoglobin to the tissues and from the alveolar gas to the haemoglobin. One of the indicators of the position of the oxygen–haemoglobin dissociation curve is the PO_2 at which haemoglobin is 50% saturated with oxygen. This point is called P50 and is normally around 3.6 kPa. Factors which shift the oxygen–haemoglobin dissociation curve to the left include:

- alkalosis
- hyperthermia
- reduced 2,3, DPG
- foetal haemoglobin
- reduced carbon dioxide.

Factors which shift the curve to the right include:

- acidosis
- hyperthermia
- increased 2,3,DPG (as in anaemia)
- hypercarbia.

Carbon dioxide

Each 100 ml of arterial blood carries 48 ml of carbon dioxide in solution, as bicarbonate, or as carbamino compounds.

AUTONOMIC NERVOUS SYSTEM – PHYSIOLOGY

Centrally, the sites of the autonomic nervous system (the hypothalamus, medulla oblongata and pons) are involved in the regulation of blood pressure, respiration, temperature and stress responses. Peripherally, the autonomic nervous system is divided into the sympathetic and parasympathetic nervous system.

SYMPATHETIC NERVOUS SYSTEM

The sympathetic nerve fibres arise from thoracolumbar segments of spinal cord (T1–L2). The pre-ganglionic fibres enter paravertebral sympathetic chains which lie lateral to the spinal cord. The post-ganglionic neurons travel to various organs in the body.

PARASYMPATHETIC NERVOUS SYSTEM

The parasympathetic neurons are located in discrete brain stem nuclei and in the sacral spinal cord. The pre-ganglionic fibres leave the brain stem via cranial nerves III, VII, IX and X and the sacral spinal cord via the pelvic nerves (S2–S4). The majority of the cranial parasympathetic outflow (75%) is contained in the vagus nerve which supplies all organs in the thorax and abdomen down to the transverse colon. Pre-ganglionic fibres of the parasympathetic nervous system travel uninterrupted to ganglions situated in or near the effector organs.

NEUROTRANSMITTERS

The primary neurotransmitter substances of the autonomic nervous system are acetylcholine and norepinephrine. Nerve fibres that secrete acetylcholine are called cholinergic and those secreting norepinephrine are called adrenergic.

- All pre-ganglionic fibres of the sympathetic and parasympathetic nervous system are cholinergic.
- All post-ganglionic parasympathetic fibres are cholinergic.

- All post-ganglionic sympathetic fibres are adrenergic, except those supplying the sweat glands which are cholinergic.

RECEPTORS

Cholinergic receptors

The cholinergic receptors are subdivided into muscarinic and nicotinic receptors. The muscarinic receptors are found on all effector cells stimulated by post-ganglionic parasympathetic nerves (for example eyes, heart, lung, bladder, gut). Nicotinic receptors are found at the autonomic ganglion (the synapse between the pre-ganglionic and post-ganglionic fibres of both sympathetic and parasympathetic nerves), and at the skeletal muscle neuromuscular junction.

Adrenergic receptors

These are divided into α and β receptors. These are further subdivided into $\alpha1$, $\alpha2$ and $\beta1$, $\beta2$ receptors.

ACTIONS OF THE AUTONOMIC NERVOUS SYSTEM

Most organs are dominantly controlled by one of the two systems. Both sympathetic as well as parasympathetic nervous systems can have excitatory as well as inhibitory effects on different organs. Sometimes the two divisions can act opposite to each other on the same organ. The overall effects of sympathetic and parasympathetic nervous stimulation of different organs are summarized in Table 1.10.

DRUGS ACTING ON THE AUTONOMIC NERVOUS SYSTEM

A variety of drugs can influence autonomic nervous system activity by acting either at autonomic ganglion, at receptor sites by promoting the release of neurotransmitters, or by blocking their actions.

Sympathomimetic drugs

The direct sympathomimetic drugs can act on α receptors or β receptors or both. Phenylephrine specifically stimulates α receptors. Dobutamine is mainly a β receptor stimulator (both $\beta1$ and $\beta2$). Dopamine and epinephrine in large doses can stimulate both α and β receptors. Certain drugs such as ephedrine and amphetamine can have sympathomimetic action by inducing the release of norepinephrine from storage vesicles.

TABLE 1.10 Actions of the autonomic nervous system

Organ	Sympathetic effects	Parasympathetic effects
Eye	Dilated pupils	Constricted pupils
Heart	Increased rate Increased conduction Increased automaticity	Bradycardia (SA node) Decreased AV node conduction
Bronchial smooth muscle	Relaxation	Contraction
Gut	Decreased motility Decreased secretions Sphincter contraction	Increased motility Increased secretions Relaxation of sphincters
Urinary bladder	Relaxation with sphincter contraction	Contraction with sphincter relaxation
Liver	Glycogenolysis and gluconeogenesis	Glycogen synthesis
Salivary gland	Increased secretions	Markedly increased secretions
Sweat glands	Increased secretions	–
Coronary blood vessels	Constriction (α) Relaxation (β)	–
Skin and mucosal blood vessels	Constriction	Relaxation
Skeletal muscle blood vessels	Constriction (α) Relaxation (β)	Relaxation

Adrenergic blocking drugs

The release of norepinephrine can be blocked by guanethidine. The receptors can be blocked by phenoxybenzamine and phentolamine (α receptor blockers) or by propranolol ($\beta1$ and $\beta2$ receptor blocker) or metoprolol ($\beta1$ receptor blocker) and other β blockers.

Cholinergic drugs

Drugs that act like acetylcholine at the effector organs are called parasympathomimetic or muscarinic drugs. These drugs either act directly on muscarinic cholinergic receptors or by prolonging the activity of acetylcholine by blocking acetylcholinesterase. Examples of these types of drugs include neostigmine, edrophonium and physostigmine.

Cholinergic blocking drugs

These drugs block the effect of acetylcholine on muscarinic types of receptors. Examples are atropine and glycopyrrolate.

ACID–BASE PHYSIOLOGY

The acid–base status of blood can be assessed by measuring the pH, $PaCO_2$ and PaO_2 of arterial blood. Changes in pH that are primarily related to changes in $PaCO_2$ are referred to as respiratory acidosis (increased $PaCO_2$) or respiratory alkalosis (decreased $PaCO_2$). Changes in pH primarily due to alterations in bicarbonate are referred to as metabolic disturbances.

Buffers

Buffers are substances which by their presence in a solution increase the amount of acid or alkali that must be added to cause a change in the pH. The buffering systems in the blood are haemoglobin, bicarbonate and plasma proteins; in interstitial fluid they are bicarbonate and phosphate; and within the cells they are proteins and phosphates.

METABOLIC ALKALOSIS

Metabolic alkalosis is diagnosed when pH is more than 7.45 and the bicarbonate concentration in plasma is more than 27 mmol/l. The causes of metabolic alkalosis are given in Table 1.11.

The consequences of metabolic alkalosis are:

- hypokalaemia
- decreased concentration of ionized calcium
- compensatory hypoventilation and CO_2 retention
- leftward shift of the oxygen–haemoglobin dissociation curve leading to reduced availability of oxygen to tissues
- decreased cardiac output.

TABLE 1.11 Causes of metabolic alkalosis

Loss of hydrogen and chloride ions in nasogastric fluid or repeated vomiting
Chronic diuretic administration
Decreased circulatory volume leading to decreased renal blood flow
Hypokalaemia

Treatment of metabolic alkalosis

- treat the underlying cause
- avoid hyperventilation
- fluid management with 0.9% saline or Hartmann's solution
- maintain renal blood flow
- potassium infusion if hypokalaemia co-exists.

METABOLIC ACIDOSIS

This is diagnosed if the pH is less than 7.35 and the bicarbonate is less than 21 mmol/l. Metabolic acidosis can occur with or without an anion gap. The commonly measured cation (sodium) usually exceeds the total concentration of anions (chlorides and bicarbonates) by 7–12 mmol/l (the anion gap).

The causes of metabolic acidosis are given in Table 1.12.

The consequences of metabolic acidosis are:

- decreased myocardial contractility leading to reduced cardiac output
- decreased systemic vascular resistance
- impaired response to inotropes
- compensatory hyperventilation
- intense sympathetic stimulation with impaired kidney and gut perfusion
- exaggerated hypotensive effects of drugs and positive pressure ventilation.

The treatment of metabolic acidosis includes:

- treatment of the primary cause such as hypotension, hypoxia or sepsis

TABLE 1.12 Causes of metabolic acidosis
With normal anion gap
Diarrhoea
Hypovolaemia
Low cardiac output
Renal failure
Hepatic failure
Sepsis
Hypothermia
With increased anion gap
Excess lactic acid or ketoacidosis
Aspirin poisoning
Ingestion of ethylene, glycol or methanol

- maintenance of compensatory hyperventilation
- sodium bicarbonate 8.4% if pH is less than 7.1.

RESPIRATORY ALKALOSIS

Respiratory alkalosis is diagnosed if the pH is more than 7.45 and $PaCO_2$ is less than 4.5 kPa. However the pH tends towards normal due to a compensatory decrease in serum bicarbonate.

Respiratory alkalosis produces:

- hypokalaemia
- hypocalcaemia
- decreased cerebral blood flow (which returns to normal over 8–24 hours corresponding to the return of CSF pH to normal).

The treatment of respiratory alkalosis is primarily the treatment of its cause (see Table 1.13).

TABLE 1.13 Causes of respiratory alkalosis

Pain
Anxiety
Hypoxia
Central nervous system disease
Systemic sepsis
Excessive IPPV

RESPIRATORY ACIDOSIS

This is diagnosed when the pH is less than 7.35 and $PaCO_2$ more than 6 kPa. Moderate increases in $PaCO_2$ are compensated by the kidneys which retain bicarbonate. Acute respiratory acidosis can be differentiated from chronic by assessing the bicarbonate concentrations. Respiratory acidosis occurs either because there is an increase in carbon dioxide production or, more commonly, there is an impairment of carbon dioxide excretion by the lungs (see Table 1.14).

Patients with chronic carbon dioxide retention require careful preoperative evaluation as they usually have advanced pulmonary disease. Often, these patients have to be cared for in intensive care or high dependency unit postoperatively and careful titration of pain control and respiratory support may be required. Administration of opioids and sedatives, even in relatively low doses, can be hazardous. Chronic respiratory acidosis is rarely amenable to treatment.

TABLE 1.14 Causes of respiratory acidosis

Impaired alveolar ventilation

Central nervous system depression (e.g. opioids, general anaesthetics)
Skeletal muscle weakness due to neuromuscular blockers or
neuromuscular disorders
Chronic obstructive pulmonary disease
Acute respiratory failure

Increased carbon dioxide production

Hypermetabolic states
Sepsis
Malignant hyperthermia

The treatment of acute respiratory acidosis includes:

- treatment of causative factors
- reversal of opioids or muscle relaxants
- mechanical ventilatory support.

AN APPROACH TO ACID–BASE INTERPRETATION

Acidosis and alkalosis can be primarily metabolic or respiratory. Metabolic disturbances are compensated by lungs; metabolic acidosis leads to hyperventilation and decreased arterial PCO_2 while alkalosis leads to hypoventilation and increased PCO_2. Respiratory disturbances are compensated by the kidneys leading to retention of bicarbonates in acidosis, and excretion of bicarbonates in alkalosis. Therefore, values of pH, $PaCO_2$ and HCO_3 in a typical blood gas analysis can be used to reach a diagnosis. The arterial blood gas results should be interpreted along with patient's history, clinical condition and electrolyte measurements.

1. Is the pH life-threatening requiring immediate intervention?
2. Is the patient breathing normally or is he/she hypo- or hyperventilating? Does the patient require ventilatory support?
3. Look at the changes in pH and the direction of change in carbon dioxide and bicarbonate concentrations:
   - An increased pH with decreased carbon dioxide and normal or reduced bicarbonates should lead to the diagnosis of respiratory alkalosis.
   - A reduced pH with raised carbon dioxide with normal or increased bicarbonate level should lead to the diagnosis of respiratory acidosis.

- A reduced pH with reduced bicarbonates and normal or reduced carbon dioxide should lead to the diagnosis of metabolic acidosis.
- An increased pH with raised bicarbonates with normal or increased carbon dioxide level should lead to the diagnosis of metabolic alkalosis.

4. Look at the associated changes in electrolytes, which may require correction, along with correction of the acid base disturbance.
5. Consider if the acid–base picture fits the clinical condition.

PHARMACOLOGY

INHALATIONAL AGENTS

Inhaled anaesthetic agents remain popular for the maintenance of anaesthesia and some may also be used for the induction of anaesthesia. Inhalational induction is the technique of choice for:

- predicted difficult airway
- difficult intravenous access
- needle phobia, including children.

The ideal inhalational agent may be described by certain characteristics (see Table 2.1). None of the currently available agents meet all these requirements.

A number of important concepts must be understood to be able to compare usefully the available agents. These are potency, minimum alveolar concentration (MAC) and blood–gas solubility. The mechanism of action of the inhaled anaesthetic agents remains unknown. However, potency which is described by the MAC value is related to lipid solubility (see Figure 2.1). The MAC value is the minimum alveolar concentration (approximated by the end-tidal concentration) of the agent that when given alone in oxygen to spontaneously breathing patients would prevent movement in 50% in response to a skin incision. It represents one easily described point on the dose–response curve and permits direct comparisons of different agents. The concentration to prevent a response in 95% of patients is approximately 1.5 MAC. In general, fractions or multiples of MAC of different agents given in combination are additive. The MAC of an agent is modified by certain factors (see Table 2.2).

The variation of MAC with age is important when comparing agents. The commonly quoted values are those determined for young adults.

TABLE 2.1 Characteristics of the ideal inhaled anaesthetic agent

A pleasant odour
Non-irritant
Low blood:gas solubility (rapid induction and recovery)
Chemically stable
Non-inflammable
Potent
Inert
Not metabolized
Non-toxic
Analgesic
Minimal depression of the cardiovascular and respiratory systems

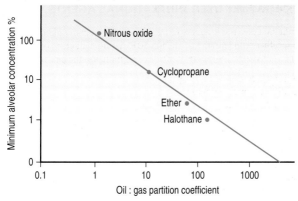

Fig. 2.1 Meyer-Overton graph. Relationship between oil solubility and potency of inhaled anaesthetic agents as described by Meyer-Overton.

TABLE 2.2 Factors which modify MAC

Increase MAC:	Decrease MAC:
CNS stimulants (e.g. amphetamines)	Sedative agents
Increased metabolism (thyrotoxicosis)	Reduced metabolism (hypothyroidism)
Reducing age (infants)	Increasing age

A number of factors increase the speed of change in the alveolar concentration (and by inference the brain concentration) of an inhaled anaesthetic agent:

- increased alveolar ventilation
- reduced cardiac output
- use of an agent with a low blood:gas solubility coefficient.

The alveolar concentration will increase more rapidly with a greater inspired concentration. In the 'overpressure' technique the inspired concentration is set to a higher level than the target required and then reduced as the target is approached. However the lowest inspired concentration is '0%' so recovery cannot be sped up this way! A lower blood:gas solubility increases the speed of reaching a new equilibrium when the inspired concentration is changed, and increases the speed at which anaesthesia can be induced during an inhalational induction and the speed of recovery when anaesthesia is discontinued.

COMMONLY USED INHALATIONAL AGENTS – TABLES 2.3 AND 2.4

The physical properties of the inhaled anaesthetic agents and the pharmacological properties of the commonly used agents are described in Tables 2.3 and 2.4 respectively.

TABLE 2.3 Physical properties of inhalational anaesthetic agents

Drug	Boiling point (°C)	MAC	Blood:gas solubility coefficient
Nitrous oxide	−89	104	0.47
Halothane	50	0.75	2.3
Enflurane	56	1.68	1.9
Isoflurane	49	1.15	1.4
Desflurane	23.9	6	0.42
Sevoflurane	58.9	2	0.69
Diethyl ether	34.6	1.92	12

TABLE 2.4 Pharmacological properties of commonly used inhalational agents

	Halothane	Isoflurane	Desflurane	Sevoflurane
Irritant	−	+	+++	−
Pungent smell	−	++	+	−
Metabolism	20%	0.17%	Virtually none	3%
Blood pressure	↓	↓↓	↑ then ↓	↓
Heart rate	↓	↑	↑ then ↓	↓
Cardiac output	↓↓	↓	↑ then ↓	↓
Arrhythmias	+ (ventricular ectopics)	−	−	−
Respiratory rate	↑	↑	↑	↑
Tidal volume	↓	↓	↓	↓
Hepatic toxicity	Rare – fatal	−	−	−
Renal toxicity	−	−	−	−
Uterine muscle tone	↓	↓	↓	↓
Cerebral autoregulation	Reduced	Preserved (at low doses)	Probably preserved at low doses	Preserved

Halothane

Halothane is used only for specific indications including inhalational induction. Fulminant hepatic failure, although rare, has led to its decline as a drug of everyday use. It may be associated with repeated use over short periods of time. Ventricular arrhythmias also limit its use.

 Repeated exposure to halothane over a short period of time may predispose to fulminant hepatic failure.

Isoflurane

Isoflurane has been used for many years and remains a satisfactory choice for maintenance of anaesthesia for the majority of cases.

Desflurane

Both sevoflurane and desflurane were introduced in the mid-1990s. Both have a low blood:gas solubility. The main advantage of desflurane is that metabolism is negligible. However, its pungency may lead to respiratory complications when first administered, which may be associated with sympathetic nervous system activation.

Sevoflurane

Suitable for inhalation induction and is more rapid than with halothane. In circle systems a potentially toxic breakdown product is produced. However, there is no evidence of toxicity in patients.

In the UK isoflurane and sevoflurane are the most frequently used agents for maintenance.

OTHER AGENTS

Enflurane

Enflurane has been superseded by more modern agents and is rarely used. One particular problem is that at moderate to high concentrations enflurane produces epileptiform paroxysmal spike activity and burst suppression on the electroencephalograph, accentuated by hypocapnia.

Diethyl ether ('ether')

Ether is flammable and can form explosive mixtures. Its high blood:gas solubility and irritant nature makes it a difficult drug to use. Salivary secretions are increased and premedication with an anti-sialogue essential. Ether stimulates ventilation in light stages of anaesthesia. There is a high incidence of postoperative nausea and vomiting. It is metabolized to water, carbon dioxide, acetaldehyde and ethanol. Although difficult to use it is considered to be a safe drug because of its high therapeutic index.

ANAESTHETIC GASES

Nitrous oxide

Nitrous oxide is a sweet-smelling, non-irritant gas. It is stored as a liquid in a cylinder at a pressure of approximately 5000 kPa. During use the cylinders should be kept vertical so that the liquid remains at the bottom. The cylinder cools as energy is used to provide the latent heat of vaporization of the liquid. Nitrous oxide is non-flammable but supports combustion. It is a weak anaesthetic (MAC = 104%) but has some analgesic properties. It is used for its analgesic properties, its low blood:gas solubility, and as a carrier gas for other agents. Its low potency means that it cannot be used as the sole anaesthetic agent and must be combined with another agent to ensure lack of awareness. It is generally considered safe and non-toxic, though this has been challenged recently (see below).

> ⚠ **As a result of differences in solubility nitrous oxide dissolves into closed air-filled spaces more rapidly than nitrogen dissolves out. This leads to an increase in pressure in spaces such as the gut, the middle ear and in a pneumothorax.**

At the end of anaesthesia nitrous oxide diffuses from the body back into the alveoli more rapidly than nitrogen diffuses from the alveolar gas into the body. This has the effect of lowering the oxygen concentration in the alveoli and may cause hypoxia (diffusion hypoxia). During recovery from nitrous oxide anaesthesia, room air should be supplemented with oxygen to prevent this. Nitrous oxide inactivates methionine synthetase. This may result in megaloblastic anaemia after prolonged nitrous oxide use. Significant changes may be seen after 6 h of use. Sub-acute combined degeneration of the cord can also occur after long-term occupational exposure. Nitrous oxide use increases the likelihood of postoperative nausea and vomiting.

Entonox

This is a 50:50 mixture of nitrous oxide and oxygen that is used for its analgesia actions – for dressing changes, field use (ambulances), and the pain of contractions during labour. It is provided pre-mixed in a cylinder and usually administered via a demand valve apparatus.

Oxygen

Oxygen is produced by the fractional distillation of air. It is stored in cylinders as a compressed gas at 13,700 kPa (137 bar) when full. Large hospitals and industrial users of oxygen store it as the liquid form in insulated tanks. Oxygen supports combustion and at high pressures it may ignite grease or oil.

Complications of long-term use of high concentrations of oxygen include:

- absorption atelectasis of the lungs and pulmonary oxygen toxicity
- retrolental fibroplasia in neonates
- carbon dioxide retention in patients with decreased chemoreceptor sensitivity to carbon dioxide
- seizure activity at hyperbaric pressures.

Medical air

Medical air is an alternative carrier gas when there is a contraindication to nitrous oxide. Most anaesthetic machines offer a choice of medical air or nitrous oxide to accompany oxygen. Compressed air is also used as a power source for medical equipment such as ventilators and surgical equipment.

Carbon dioxide

Carbon dioxide has been used to facilitate inhalational induction of anaesthesia by adding it to the inspired gases. However, this practice is used infrequently now and is no longer necessary with modern inhalational agents.

> ⚠ **Inadvertent carbon dioxide administration is dangerous and carbon dioxide cylinders should not be routinely attached to anaesthetic machines.**

INTRAVENOUS AGENTS

INTRAVENOUS ANAESTHETIC AGENTS

The most commonly used general anaesthetic technique is intravenous induction of anaesthesia followed by maintenance using inhaled agents. In addition, drugs are given to produce analgesia and muscle relaxation if necessary. Intravenous induction of anaesthesia has a number of advantages:

- speed of induction
- smooth induction
- low incidence of side-effects
- patient acceptability.

The introduction of intravenous induction agents in the middle of the 20th century revolutionized anaesthesia – partly because of the difficulty and poor patient acceptance of induction with the then available inhalational drugs such as ether (diethyl ether). Intravenous induction drugs may also be used to maintain anaesthesia in a total intravenous anaesthesia (TIVA) technique, to supplement inhalational anaesthesia, and for sedation in the intensive care unit and during procedures performed under regional anaesthesia. The characteristics of the ideal intravenous agent are given in Table 2.5.

The onset of action of an intravenous induction agent depends on the drug crossing the blood–brain barrier. The speed of injection, blood flow to the brain, lipid solubility and protein binding of the drug will affect this. Recovery from these agents is predominantly due to either redistribution from the brain to other tissues such as muscle and fat or to metabolism in the liver and other organs.

The choice of intravenous induction agent depends on assessing these factors for each patient. See Table 2.6 for a description of the properties of the commonly used intravenous agents.

Propofol

Propofol is the most commonly used intravenous induction agent. Because upper airway reflexes are inhibited soon after induction of anaesthesia it is the most suitable agent if a laryngeal mask airway is to be inserted. Induction with propofol is usually smooth and recovery is rapid. Pain on injection can be reduced by the addition of a small dose of lidocaine (lignocaine) (an unlicensed practice) or the use of a new formulation. The main disadvantage of propofol

---

TABLE 2.5 Characteristics of the ideal intravenous induction agent

A smooth and rapid onset
A rapid recovery
No pain or injection
Minimal side-effects
No toxicity

TABLE 2.6 Properties of the commonly used intravenous induction agents

	Thiopental sodium	Propofol	Etomidate
Preparation	Powder	Emulsion	In proplyene glycol
Strength	25 mg/ml (when diluted)	10 mg/ml	2 mg/ml
Irritant if extravasated	+++	+	+
Painful injection	–	+	++
Porphyria	Not safe	Probably safe	Not safe
Excitatory effects	–	+	++
Dose	3–5 mg/kg	1–2 mg/kg	0.1–0.2 mg/kg
Speed of recovery	+	++	++
Redistribution	+++	+	++
Metabolism	+	+++	++
Accumulation	+++	–	–
CVS depression	+	++	–
Apnoea	+	++	–
Nausea	+	–	++
Glucocorticoid suppression	–	+	+++
Allergic reactions	++	+	(+)

is cardiovascular depression immediately after induction. This is dose-dependent and more common in the elderly or sick patient. Propofol may have some, short-lived anti-emetic actions.

Etomidate

Etomidate is often used in patients at risk of cardiovascular collapse due to poor cardiac status or shock. However the evidence for any benefit is poor and the patient's condition should be optimized as much as possible prior to induction. Postoperative nausea and delirium can be difficult to manage.

Thiopental sodium (thiopentone)

Thiopental remains popular with some anaesthetists when the trachea is to be intubated. The risk of anaphylactoid reactions is greatest with this drug compared with the other agents. Extravasation injuries can cause major morbidity.

Ketamine

Ketamine is unlike other intravenous induction agents. It produces a dissociative state. Patients may have their eyes open, but it is not possible to communicate with them and they have no recall. It is a very effective analgesic. Its main advantages are that it is associated with myocardial stimulation leading to preservation of cardiac output and a rise in blood pressure and heart rate; it may be given intramuscularly and intravenously; and airways reflexes are better preserved than with other agents (although a patent airway cannot be guaranteed). Its main disadvantages are that its use is associated with postoperative nightmares and it increases cerebral blood flow and intracranial pressure. Nausea and vomiting is frequent and excess salivation occurs. It is supplied as a 1, 5 or 10% solution. The usual intravenous dose is 1–2 mg/kg (10 mg/kg intramuscularly). A single dose will last for 5–10 minutes and repeated doses or an infusion may be used to maintain anaesthesia. It is used in shocked patients, as an analgesic/sedative to position patients prior to regional blockade, when intravenous access is problematic and as a field agent.

MAINTENANCE OF ANAESTHESIA

The ideal intravenous agent for the maintenance of anaesthesia has predictable pharmacokinetics, few side-effects, and an absence of accumulation on prolonged use. Manual infusion schemes can be used to administer the correct quantity of drug to produce the desired depth of anaesthesia, but a microprocessor controlled pump to produce a 'predicted plasma concentration' of agent has been developed. These pumps use population based pharmacokinetic models to simplify the complicated infusion schemes necessary to take into account the initial bolus, the redistribution of the drug from the blood and the brain to other compartments, and the clearance from the plasma (due to continuing redistribution and elimination from the body). The only agent currently available that is suitable for total intravenous anaesthesia (TIVA) is propofol. The Target Controlled Infusion (TCI) system, marketed by one pharmaceutical company, uses pharmacokinetic data programmed into specially made pumps to provide such an infusion scheme.

ADJUVANTS

Other drugs may be used to supplement the intravenous induction agents particularly at the time of induction. This technique is known as co-induction. Advantages may include a 'smoother' induction and reduction of side-effects. The opioids may be used for co-induction and are considered elsewhere. The other major group is the benzodiazepines. The α_2 agonist dexmedetomidine may be available soon as an adjuvant agent.

Benzodiazepines

The benzodiazpeines are agonists at GABA receptors. They are anxiolytic, sedative, and produce amnesia (antegrade) (see Table 2.7). As well as being used for co-induction these agents may also be used alone for their sedative properties. In large doses they may be used to induce anaesthesia; however, they suppress respiration and may depress the cardiovascular system. They reduce muscle spasm and are anticonvulsant. Benzodiazepines may be given by a variety of routes, and the main differences in the available agents are pharmacokinetic. In general, their duration of action is longer than the commonly used intravenous induction agents. Flumazenil is a specific antagonist at the GABA receptor.

TABLE 2.7 Properties of the commonly used benzodiazepines

Drug	Use	Dose	Notes
Midazolam	Co-induction	0.3 mg/kg	Oral preparation available in some countries.
	Sedation	0.01–0.1 mg/kg	Duration ~1 h
Diazepam	Premedication	0.1–0.2 mg/kg	Onset of action 30 min after p.o. administration.
	Sedative and anticonvulsant	0.05–0.2 mg/kg	Duration up to 4 h.
Temazepam	Premedication	10–30 mg	Duration ~ 4–6 h
Lorazepam	Premedication	1–3 mg	Duration up to 24 h.

ANALGESIC DRUGS

The analgesic drugs used for intraoperative and postoperative use are the simple analgesics, the non-steroidal anti-inflammatory drugs, and the opioids. Local anaesthetics and nitrous oxide are also analgesic drugs and are considered elsewhere in this chapter.

SIMPLE ANALGESICS

Paracetamol is termed a simple analgesic although its exact mode and site of action are unknown. It is also used as an antipyretic.

Although only a mild analgesic it is devoid of side-effects (except when excess doses are taken when it may result in fulminant hepatic failure). Paracetamol is used for pain relief after minor operations such as body surface surgery. It is often used in combination with NSAIDs, and with weak or strong opioids for mild to moderate pain after more major surgery.

NON-STEROIDAL ANTI-INFLAMMATORY DRUGS (NSAID)

These agents are useful for mild-to-moderate pain, and have an opioid-sparing effect when used for more severe pain. They may also be combined with paracetamol. There are a large number of these agents although those used frequently in the perioperative period are ibuprofen, diclofenac and ketorolac. Aspirin is not used for acute pain therapy because of a high incidence of side-effects. NSAIDs have widespread actions mostly due to inhibition of cyclo-oxygenase leading to reduced prostaglandin, prostacyclin and thromboxane synthesis. They exert most of their analgesic action peripherally but may also have a direct, central analgesic action. In addition to analgesia these drugs are anti-pyretic and have an anti-platelet action. Side-effects of NSAIDs include:

- damaged gastrointestinal mucosa
- reduced renal blood flow
- bronchospasm
- bleeding.

 Bronchospasm may occur in asthmatic patients and those with nasal polyps are at increased risk.

The side-effects limit the use of these drugs. In particular, they are not recommended immediately after major surgery when fluid balance disturbances may have already reduced splanchnic and renal blood flow. Many anaesthetists also avoid their use in patients with a history of peptic ulceration or reflux oesophagitis. There are two types of cyclo-oxygenase (COX) – 1 and 2. Analgesic actions appear to be mediated via COX 2, while the main side-effects are mediated via COX 1. In theory the use of specific inhibitors of COX 2 such as parecoxib will limit side-effects.

Ibuprofen and diclofenac are available orally, diclofenac is also available as a suppository and for intramuscular injection. Ketorolac can be given intravenously but should not be used intraoperatively. An intravenous preparation of parecoxib (a COX 2 inhibitor) is now available for use in acute pain, but the proposed benefits of these agents have not been convincingly demonstrated and there is a suggestion that other side-effects such as cardiovascular morbidity and mortality may be increased with their long-term use.

OPIOIDS

Opioids have a number of actions that can be useful to anaesthetists – analgesia, increasing the depth of anaesthesia, sedation, anxiolysis and cough suppression (see Table 2.8). Although all opioids are active at μ (mu) receptors some are also active at other receptors such as δ (delta) and κ (kappa). Some are partial agonists at the μ receptor and some have mixed agonist and antagonist action at different opioid receptors. The other differences in their actions are mostly pharmacokinetic. Analgesia is mediated through receptors in the central grey matter of the brain stem and the substantia gelatinosa of the spinal cord. The onset of action of the analgesic action is related to the lipid solubility of the different agents. The more lipid soluble agents also tend to have a shorter duration of action because they redistribute to other tissues.

TABLE 2.8 Actions of opioid agonists

CNS	Reduced anxiety, awareness, pain, and respiratory drive, increased vomiting, papillary constriction, ADH release, vagally mediated bradycardia Tolerance, tachyphylaxis, dependence
Smooth muscle	Decreased peristalsis, increased tone Vasodilatation Bronchoconstriction Biliary sphincter spasm

The analgesic actions of the opioids are most effective against dull, continuous visceral pain. The psychological component of pain is also reduced. Respiratory depression (reduced respiratory rate) is the most important side-effect. Nausea and vomiting are common, as is urinary retention and generalized itch. Opioids can be given by a number of routes including intravenous, subcutaneous, intramuscular, orally, and into the epidural and subarachnoid spaces. Fentanyl may be given also transdermally. The usual route of administration is parenteral with intravenous bolus doses, continuous infusions, and patient controlled analgesia (PCA) systems used.

Morphine

The onset of action after intravenous administration of morphine is 5–10 min, with a duration of action of 2–4 h. After oral administration the onset of action is about 1 h and there is significant first-pass metabolism. A slow-release preparation is available. Morphine is conjugated in the liver to morphine-6-glucuronide, an active metabolite, which is excreted by the kidneys.

Diamorphine

Diamorphine is the diacetyl ester analogue of morphine. It is more fat-soluble and consequently has a faster onset of action. It is approximately twice as potent as morphine.

Pethidine

Pethidine has one-tenth of the potency of morphine but is otherwise similar. It may cause less increase in smooth muscle tone and also has some anti-cholinergic and local anaesthetic actions. It may cause severe reactions in patients also receiving monoamine oxidase inhibitors. A metabolite – norpethidine– may accumulate in patients with renal impairment and cause convulsions.

The usual starting dose for intravenous bolus injection of these agents when used for acute pain is:

● morphine: 0.05–0.1 mg/kg
● diamorphine: 0.025–0.05 mg/kg
● pethidine: 0.5–1.0 mg/kg.

The short-acting derivatives of pethidine (fentanyl, alfentanil and remifentanil) are usually used intraoperatively only (see Table 2.9).

Fentanyl

Fentanyl is 100 times more potent than morphine. It has a rapid onset of action (1–2 min), and a short duration (20 min) predominantly due to redistribution. High doses may lead to accumulation

TABLE 2.9 Bolus dose and infusion rates for the short-acting opioids		
	Bolus dose (for co-induction)	Infusion rate
Fentanyl	1–2 µg/kg	Not suitable
Alfentanil	5–10 µg/kg	0.5–1 µg/kg/min
Remifentanil	0.25–1 µg/kg	0.125–1 µg/kg/min

and prolonged action. Fentanyl has very little effect on the cardio-vascular system apart from vagally-induced bradycardia. However, large doses may lead to chest wall rigidity that may impair ventilation. Fentanyl may be infused into the epidural space in combination with a local anaesthetic for postoperative analgesia.

Alfentanil
Alfentanil is more lipid-soluble with a faster onset of action than fentanyl. It has a short elimination half-life, and is suitable for use as an infusion.

Remifentanil
Remifentanil is very lipid soluble with a rapid onset, and a very short elimination half life. It is suitable for infusion and the half-life is not affected by the duration of infusion. It is metabolized by non-specific plasma and tissue esterases. It is often used to replace nitrous oxide as the analgesic component of balanced general anaesthesia. Because of its very short duration of action another longer-acting analgesic is invariably required after remifentanil is stopped.

Codeine phosphate
Codeine phosphate causes less respiratory depression than morphine but also has much less analgesic action. To act it must be converted to morphine, and the speed of this reaction is highly variable between different individuals. Because there is less first pass metabolism than with other opioids it can be used orally. It is used most frequently in neuroanaesthetic and paediatric practice, probably because it is perceived to have a high safety margin. This also means that it is a poor analgesic in the doses commonly used. It is, however, a good cough suppressant.

Dihydrocodeine
Similar to codeine but more potent, dihydrocodeine is used for mild-to-moderate pain. It is effective orally and is often used when morphine is no longer needed.

Tramadol
Tramadol has weak agonist activity at opioid receptors. It is also active against noradrenergic and 5-hydroxytryptamine pathways. It may be given orally or intravenously, and is used as an alternative to morphine in PCA systems. Its duration of action is 3–6h. It is most commonly used orally as an alternative to dihydrocodeine for mild-to-moderate pain. There is some evidence that its use intraoperatively may increase the likelihood of awareness.

Partial agonists and mixed agonists/antagonists

These groups include buprenorphine, pentazocine, nalbuphine and meptazinol. These agents have, in general, not successfully replaced morphine or pethidine because of a variety of side-effects.

Naloxone

Naloxone is a μ receptor antagonist. It is used to overcome the side-effects of opioids, in particular respiratory depression and excess sedation. The usual dose is 0.1–0.4 mg i.v. It has a short duration of action (about 1 h) compared with morphine and recurrence of the side-effects is likely. Repeat doses or an infusion of naloxone may be necessary and patients should be observed in a postoperative recovery room or HDU area.

LOCAL ANAESTHETICS

Local anaesthetic drugs act by producing a reversible block to the transmission of a nerve impulse in a peripheral nerve. Although a number of drug types have local anaesthetic properties, those currently used specifically for the purpose of nerve blockade are all derived from cocaine. These agents are very similar chemically and contain either an amide or an ester intermediate chain linking an aromatic group to an amine group. They act by crossing the cell membrane to enter the cell, blocking the sodium channels and, therefore, blocking membrane depolarization. They act on sodium channels in all excitable tissues. The actions are concentration dependent and as the drug is cleared from plasma it diffuses from the site of injection in to the blood.

Ester local anaesthetics are broken down rapidly by plasma cholinesterases. The amide local anaesthetics are metabolized in the liver and the rate of clearance is dependent on liver blood flow. Severe hepatic dysfunction slows amide metabolism and abnormal or reduced cholinesterase level slows ester metabolism.

TOXICITY

See Action Plan 21.

The toxicity of local anaesthetics results from high concentrations in the systemic circulation and the agents reaching the heart and brain where the same membrane stabilizing properties depress the function of these organs. The early signs of CNS toxicity are:

- tingling on the tongue
- tingling around the mouth

- light-headedness
- anxiety.

These signs are followed by drowsiness and then coma and convulsions. Cardiovascular toxicity results in myocardial depression and vasodilatation. Bupivacaine toxicity is associated with ventricular fibrillation that may be resistant to cardioversion. Convulsions are treated with diazepam or thiopental, and cardiovascular collapse is treated with a sympathomimetic agent such as ephedrine or epinephrine. Local anaesthetic drugs may also cause anaphylactoid reactions. These are usually due to ester local anaesthetics, and such reactions to amides are very rare. Skin reactions to ester agents are also common.

Systemic toxicity is usually due to inadvertent intravascular injection, but may also be due to overdosage. Overdosage depends on the site of injection as absorption from a vascular site such as the intercostal space is much more rapid than from a relatively avascular region such as the skin (after infiltration anaesthesia). Rapid absorption results in high peak plasma levels, whereas slower absorption allows time for metabolism as the drug enters the systemic circulation. The sites of rapid absorption of local anaesthetics are:

- intercostal space
- epidural space
- brachial plexus
- sites of the lower limb major nerve blocks.

Absorption from the site of injection may be reduced by use of vasoconstrictors (such as epinephrine) added to the local anaesthetic solution. In intravenous regional anaesthesia (IVRA or Bier's block), the tourniquet is released after a period of time has elapsed to allow the drug to bind to proteins in the tissues. If the tourniquet is released prematurely then very high plasma concentrations can ensue leading to toxicity. Prevention of toxicity depends on careful use to avoid accidental intravascular injection. Aspiration prior to injection and repeat aspiration after every 5–10 ml of injection may reduce the incidence of this complication but will not prevent it altogether. Although the maximum doses of the commonly used local anaesthetics are published (see Table 2.10), these do not usually take into account the differing rates of absorption from different injection sites.

> ⚠ **Facilities for resuscitation (airway maintenance, intermittent positive pressure ventilation, oxygen source, circulatory support equipment and resuscitation drugs) must be available wherever local anaesthetics are used.**

TABLE 2.10 Maximum doses of commonly available local anaesthetics

Drug	Without epinephrine	With epinephrine
Lidocaine (lignocaine)	3 mg/kg	7 mg/kg
Bupivacaine	2 mg/kg	2 mg/kg
L-bupivacaine	2 mg/kg	2 mg/kg
Ropivacaine	3.5 mg/kg	3.5 mg/kg
Prilocaine	6 mg/kg	9 mg/kg

ESTER LOCAL ANAESTHETICS

Cocaine
No longer used by anaesthetists because of its toxicity and potential for abuse, cocaine is still used by ENT surgeons to 'anaesthetize' the nose. The main advantage is its marked vasoconstrictor action which reduces bleeding from the nasal mucosa. It is a marked central nervous and cardiovascular system stimulant.

Benzocaine
Used for topical anaesthesia.

Amethocaine
Used for topical anaesthesia only. A 4% gel preparation with a rapid onset of analgesia (30 min) is used to anaesthetize the skin prior to intravenous cannula insertion. A 1% solution is used to anaesthetize the conjunctiva.

AMIDE LOCAL ANAESTHETICS

Lidocaine (lignocaine)
Lidocaine is a relatively safe agent used routinely for all types of local and regional blockade. Its onset of action is rapid, but its relatively short duration of action is a disadvantage. It is used topically (4%) to anaesthetize the upper airway prior to an awake intubation, for infiltration anaesthesia (0.5–1%), and for epidural and peripheral nerve block (1–2% solutions). Lidocaine is also used intravenously as an antiarrhythmic agent.

Prilocaine
Less toxic than lidocaine and used for IVRA in the UK. However, metabolism results in a metabolite that may cause methaemoglobinaemia if large doses are used. Fetal haemoglobin is particularly sensitive and prilocaine should not be used in labouring women.

Bupivacaine
Bupivacaine has a longer duration of action than lidocaine. It is the standard drug for many procedures such as peripheral nerve blockade, epidural and subarachnoid blockade. The usual concentrations used are 0.25 and 0.5%. A 0.75% solution is available but should not be used for epidural anaesthesia following reports of cardiovascular collapse. Concerns about cardiovascular toxicity (see above) limit its use in high quantities. A hyperbaric 0.5% solution of bupivacaine is available for subarachnoid use.

L-bupivacaine
L-bupivacaine is one of the stereoisomers of bupivacaine that has less cardiovascular toxicity than the parent drug. The dosage and use are otherwise identical.

Ropivacaine
Ropivacaine is very similar to bupivacaine, but slightly less potent and with a slightly shorter duration of action.

Eutetic mixture of local anaesthetics (EMLA)
This is a mixture of the base forms of prilocaine and lidocaine that is formulated as a cream and used to provide topical anaesthesia for venepuncture after 1 h.

AGENTS USED TO MODIFY BLOCK

The action of local anaesthetics may be modified by the addition of other agents (see Table 2.11).

> ⚠ **Vasoconstrictors should not be used when the local anaesthetic is to be used near an end-artery such as in the penis or the digital arteries supplying the fingers and toes because of the risk of ischaemia.**

TABLE 2.11 Local anaesthetic adjuvants

Agent	Action
Vasoconstrictors: epinephrine (1 in 200,000) felypressin	More intense block Prolong duration Reduce toxicity
Sodium bicarbonate	Increase speed of onset
Hyaluronidase	Aid spread of local anaesthetic drug

NEUROMUSCULAR BLOCKING AGENTS (MUSCLE RELAXANTS)

These drugs are used to block neuromuscular conduction at the motor end-plate. There are two groups – the depolarizing and the non-depolarizing agents (see Table 2.12). They were first introduced in the 1940s to provide complete muscle paralysis and facilitate tracheal intubation. However, some degree of muscle relaxation can also be achieved by the use of inhalational agents and tracheal intubation can be achieved under deep inhalational anaesthesia alone. Local or regional muscle paralysis can also be achieved by the use of local anaesthetics.

The normal physiological process at the neuromuscular junction is for acetylcholine to be released from the presynaptic nerve ending as the result of the passage of a nerve impulse down the nerve fibre. The acetylcholine crosses the synaptic cleft and interacts with nicotinic acetylcholine receptors concentrated around the mouths of the junctional folds in the postsynaptic membrane of the motor end-plate. The acetylcholine receptors in the motor end-plate consist of five sub-units, two of which interact with acetylcholine. The result of the interaction is to lead to a structural change in the receptor and the opening of an ion channel. An inward movement of sodium and calcium ions and an outward movement of potassium ions leads to depolarization and then muscular contraction.

The acetylcholine is broken down (hydrolysed) by acetylcholinesterase present in the synaptic cleft. The release of acetylcholine is under the control of positive feedback action of acetylcholine

TABLE 2.12 Comparison of depolarizing and non-depolarizing block		
	Depolarizing block	Non-depolarizing (competitive) block
Muscle fasciculations	Prior to establishment of block	None
Fade	None	On repeated stimulation
Post-tetanic facilitation	None	Present
Effect of anticholinesterase	Block potentiated	Block reversed
Repeat doses	Block changed to non-depolarizing type of block (but not reversible)	Summative effects

itself on pre-junctional receptors on the nerve terminal. There is a wide safety margin and up to 70% of post-junctional receptors are redundant – and can be blocked before clinical muscle weakness is seen. Extrajunctional postsynaptic receptors can develop along the muscle fibre in certain disease states (see below). These extrajunctional receptors are more sensitive to depolarizing relaxants and among other actions cause an exaggerated release of potassium from the muscle fibre cells. The non-depolarizing agents are competitive antagonists at the nicotinic receptor. Depolarizing agents mimic the action of acetylcholine on the postsynaptic receptor but remain bound to the receptor preventing any other neuromuscular transmission.

DEPOLARIZING NEUROMUSCULAR BLOCKING AGENTS

Succinylcholine (suxamethonium)

This is the only depolarizing agent available for clinical use in the UK. The molecule has two quaternary ammonium radicals which bind to the acetylcholine receptor resulting in prolonged ion-channel opening. Succinylcholine causes an initial depolarization followed by a prolonged relaxation resistant to further stimulation. The normal intubation dose of succinylcholine (1–1.5 mg/kg) results in full relaxation after 60 seconds. It may be given intra-muscularly in exceptional circumstances (e.g. into the tongue). It is used predominantly when a rapid onset of neuromuscular blockade is required – for example with a suspected full stomach. It also has the shortest duration of action making it suitable if a difficult intubation is predicted.

> ⚠ **Recovery from suxamethonium takes between 5 and 10 minutes and if intubation is not achieved, hypoxia will develop before recovery occurs if the patient's lungs are not ventilated.**

Recovery from succinylcholine blockade occurs because of metabolism of the drug by plasma cholinesterase in the plasma. A small amount of the drug is excreted unchanged by the kidney. Abnormalities of plasma cholinesterase can lead to prolonged action (see Action Plan 30).

Succinylcholine has a number of side-effects limiting its use (see Table 2.13).

TABLE 2.13 Side-effects of succinylcholine

Side-effect	Comment
Muscle pains (myalgia)	Common in young, fit patients Reduced by prior administration of a small dose of a non-depolarizing agent
Increased intraocular pressure	Shortlasting Theoretical risk of expulsion of the contents of the eye with an open eye injury
Increased intragastric pressure	Counterbalanced by increase in tone in the lower oesophageal sphincter
Hyperkalaemia	Rise of 0.5 mmol/L in healthy patients Greater rise in presence of extrajunctional acetylcholine receptors: burns patients, muscular dystrophies, dystrophia myotonica, spastic parapesis
Muscarinic effects	Bradycardia after a second or subsequent doses
Malignant hyperthermia	
Anaphylactoid reactions	

NON-DEPOLARIZING NEUROMUSCULAR BLOCKING AGENTS

These drugs are competitive antagonists at the nicotinic postsynaptic acetylcholine receptor. At the end of the surgical procedure no further relaxant is given and the drug diffuses away from the receptor and into the plasma from where it is cleared. An anticholinesterase agent given at this time antagonizes acetylcholinesterase and increases the amount of acetylcholine available at the motor end-plate to overcome any remaining receptor occupancy. There are two main groups – the benzylisoquinoliniums and the aminosteroids.

Benzylisoquinoliniums

These agents are related to the first non-depolarizing agent to enter clinical use – tubocurare – which is no longer in use. Many are associated with release of histamine (see Table 2.14). Atracurium and cisatracurium (one of the isomers in atracurium) are broken down by Hofmann degradation. This is a phenomenon in which spontaneous breakdown occurs in the plasma in a reaction that is pH and temperature-dependent but does not require an enzyme or organ

TABLE 2.14 Characteristics of the benzylisoquiniliniums

	Atracurium	Cisatracurium	Mivacurium	Doxacurium*
Intubating dose (mg/kg)	0.5	0.15	0.15–0.2	0.03–0.05
Onset time (min)	2–3	3	3	4–6
Duration (min)	30–40	30–40	15–25	60–120
Histamine release	+	–	++	–
Renal excretion	–	–	–	–
Hofmann degradation	+	+	–	–
Ester hydrolysis	–	–	+	–

*Not available in the UK.

system. These two drugs do not accumulate in renal or hepatic failure. One of the breakdown products (laudanosine) is epileptogenic, but the quantity produced in clinical use results in a plasma concentration much less than that shown to be associated with seizure production.

Mivacurium is metabolized by plasma cholinesterase. Spontaneous recovery is rapid and an anticholinesterase is not required. However, abnormalities of plasma cholinesterase will also prolong the duration of action of this drug.

Doxacurium is a long-acting agent not available in the UK.

Aminosteroids

In general these agents produce fewer cardiovascular side-effects than the benzylisoquiniliniums, and less histamine release. Pancuronium and to a lesser extent rocuronium cause tachycardia secondary to a vagolytic action. Pancuronium also has some sympathomimetic actions. They are excreted by the kidney, with some hepatic metabolism and secretion into the bile contributing to their clearance (see Table 2.15).

Anticholinesterases

These agents are used to increase the amount of acetylcholine available at the motor end-plate to overcome the competitive block of the acetylcholine receptors by non-depolarizing muscle relaxants. They act by inhibiting acetylcholinesterase. Only neostigmine is used clinically in anaesthesia. Anticholinesterases act at all cholinergic receptors (nicotinic and muscarinic) and it is necessary to block the action at the muscarinic receptors with an anticholinergic such as atropine or glycopyrrolate to prevent bradycardia,

TABLE 2.15 Characteristics of the aminosteroids

	Vecuronium	Rocuronium	Pancuronium	Pipecuronium*
Intubation dose (mg/kg)	0.1	0.6	0.1	0.07
Onset time (min)	3	1–1½	3–4	5
Duration (min)	30–40	30–40	60–90	60–120
Vagolytic	–	+	+	–
Renal excretion	+	+	++	++
Biliary secretion	++	++	+	(+)

*Not available in the UK.

salivation, sweating, bronchospasm, increased gut motility and blurred vision. Anticholinesterases are also used orally to treat myasthenia gravis.

The usual dose of neostigmine is 2.5–5 mg, combined with atropine 1.2 mg or glycopyrrolate 0.5 mg. The onset time is about 2 min with a peak effect at 5–7 min.

Non-depolarizing blockade should only be reversed if there is some evidence of spontaneous recovery – for example if the first and second twitch to a train-of-four stimulation can be detected (see Chapter 5). Adequate recovery has occurred if the train-of-four ratio is 0.7 or greater. If non-depolarizing blockade is not adequately reversed muscle weakness can continue after the patient has regained consciousness.

Signs of partial reversal of neuromuscular block are:

- Shallow respiration
- Jerky movements of limbs and inability to lift head and protrude tongue
- Restlessness
- Double vision.

This may be both distressing for the patient and lead to inadequate respiration and inability to maintain a patent airway and protect the upper airway from aspiration. The usual treatment is to give another dose of the anticholinesterase while reassuring the patient and maintaining adequate ventilation.

PHYSICS

An understanding of certain principles of physics is essential for the safe use of many pieces of anaesthetic equipment including the anaesthesia machine and monitoring devices. The SI system is now used universally with only a small number of exceptions, the commonest of which is the use of millimetres of mercury (mmHg) to measure arterial blood pressure.

GASES

A gas expands to occupy the total space of the container in which it is in. There are three important laws that describe the behaviour of gases:

Boyle's Law: At a constant temperature, the volume (V) of a given mass of gas is inversely proportional to its pressure (P) (PV = k).

Charles' Law: At a constant pressure, the volume of a given mass of gas is proportional to its temperature (T) (V = kT).

Gay-Lussac's Law: At a constant volume, the pressure of a given mass of gas is proportional to its temperature (P = kT).

One other important principle is that in a mixture of gases the pressure exerted by each gas is the same as if that gas was alone in the container (Dalton's Law).

If the temperature of a gas is reduced it will form a liquid (i.e. when the temperature is below the boiling point). A gas can also be liquefied by increasing the pressure, provided the temperature is below the 'critical temperature'. This is the temperature above which a gas cannot be liquefied irrespective of the pressure applied. The critical temperatures of oxygen and air are well below room temperature (see Table 3.1), therefore cylinders of these gases only contain compressed gas and not liquid.

Large refrigerated containers of oxygen are used to store oxygen at hospitals. The liquefied state is possible because the tem-

TABLE 3.1 Critical temperature of commonly used anaesthetic 'gases'

Gas	Critical temperature
Oxygen	−118.0 °C
Nitrous oxide	36.5 °C
Carbon dioxide	31.0 °C
Air	−141.0 °C
Entonox	−7.0 °C

perature is maintained below the critical temperature. As oxygen and air cylinders contain only gas, the volume of gas in the cylinder is proportional to the pressure in the cylinder (Boyle's Law). The critical temperatures of nitrous oxide and carbon dioxide are above room temperature. Therefore, cylinders of these gases will contain both the liquid and the gaseous form. The pressure in these cylinders remains constant until all the liquid has vaporized and only gas remains. The pressure will then reduce as the remaining gas is used. In most hospitals nitrous oxide is stored centrally in a group or bank of cylinders known as a manifold.

A gas stored under pressure as a liquid must be provided with a gas filled space above the liquid to permit expansion of the liquid if the temperature of the cylinder increases. Therefore, even when 'full' these cylinders have a gas space above the liquid. As gas is drawn off the cylinder the temperature will fall due to the energy used as the liquid vaporizes (latent heat of vaporization). The outside of the cylinder may develop ice around it as the cylinder cools below room temperature.

A mixture of oxygen and nitrous oxide in equal proportions is often known by its tradename – Entonox. The presence of the oxygen reduces the critical temperature of nitrous oxide to −7°C and at room temperature the mixture is a gas. Below −7°C the nitrous oxide liquefies and any gas drawn off will be predominantly oxygen. As the oxygen is used up the gas being drawn off becomes predominantly nitrous oxide with the possibility that a hypoxic gas will be delivered.

> ⚠️ **Entonox cylinders must be stored above the critical temperature and if recently rewarmed from a colder temperature, should be inverted several times before use to mix the gases in the cylinder.**

PRESSURE

Pressure is force per unit area. The SI unit of pressure is the Pascal which is defined as a force of 1 newton acting over 1 square metre. The units commonly used are kilopascal (kPa) and 100 kPa is the same as 1 bar (approximately one atmosphere at sea level).

If a similar force is exerted on the plunger of two syringes, the pressure generated will be greater in a small syringe (for example a 2 ml syringe) than a larger syringe (for example a 20 ml syringe) because of the smaller surface area in the small syringe.

The simplest form of pressure measurement device is a fluid-filled manometer where the height of the column of fluid is equal to the pressure exerted on the column (Figure 3.1). For gases at higher pressures an aneroid (bellows) gauge (Figure 3.2) or Bourdon tube gauge are used. In these devices an increase in pressure in a hollow metal chamber distorts the chamber's shape causing an indicator to move along a calibrated scale. Pressure in liquids is usually measured either with a manometer or by displacement of a membrane forming part of an electronic transducer. A transducer converts energy of one type to another. In this case the potential energy from the pressure in the liquid is converted to electrical energy. A manometer can be filled with any fluid. However, the more dense the fluid the greater the pressure that can be measured. In anaesthetic practice pressures up to one atmosphere are usually described as the height of the equivalent water (cmH_2O) or mercury (mmHg) manometer column:

$$7.5\,mmHg = 10.2\,cmH_2O = 1\,kPa$$

The pressure of gas in cylinders is much higher than can be safely connected to a patient circuit via an anaesthetic machine and so a pressure-reducing valve must be used (Figure 3.3). Gas

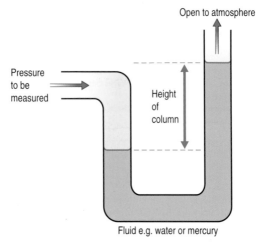

Fig. 3.1 Simple manometer – the height of column is proportional to the applied pressure.

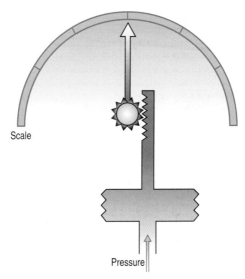

Fig. 3.2 Aneroid manometer to measure pressure in gas cylinders and pipelines.

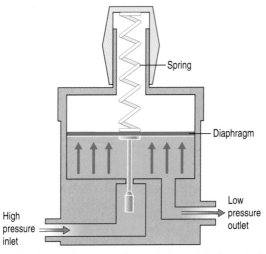

Fig. 3.3 Valve to reduce pressure in gas cylinders and pipelines prior to entering the anaesthetic machine.

entering via the high pressure inlet raises the diaphragm and causes the valve in the inlet chamber to close. By increasing the force that the spring exerts on the diaphragm, the pressure which raises the diaphragm increases and the outlet pressure rises.

GAS VOLUMES

Gas volumes are measured with a spirometer. In anaesthesia a Wright's respirometer is used. This is an anenometer – where the passage of gas through a chamber causes rotation of a vane. The number or rotations is proportional to the volume of gas passing through the chamber. An electronic version in which the measurement is automatically integrated to provide details of both volume and flow is available.

FLOW

Flow is the movement of a volume of fluid (gas or liquid) past a point in a given time. In a tube, flow may be either laminar or turbulent. In laminar flow, the flow is smooth without eddies or turbulence. The flow is fastest at the centre of the tube and slowest (approaching zero) at the sides of the tube. The flow is proportional to the pressure difference between the two ends of the tube. The effect of changes to the radius of the tube on laminar flow is large as it is the 4th power of the radius that determines flow.

The Hagen–Poiseuille equation describes laminar flow through a tube:

$$\text{Flow} = \pi P r^4 / 8nl$$

where: P is the pressure across the tube; r its radius; n the viscosity of the fluid; l the length of the tube.

Turbulent flow usually occurs when the velocity of the fluid increases. In this situation the flow is inversely proportional to the density and proportional to the square of the radius. The resistance to flow varies with the magnitude of the flow. The corrugations found in the tubing of most anaesthetic circuits decrease the velocity at which turbulent flow occurs. In addition sharp bends such as those found in angle-pieces induce turbulent flow.

Most anaesthetic machines have a mechanical method for regulating and indicating gas flow. The most common is the variable orifice flowmeter (or Rotameter) (Figure 3.4). This is a tapered tube, which widens as it ascends. Gas flow exerts a force on the bobbin and the mass of the bobbin is supported by this force. As

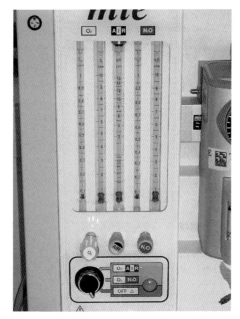

Fig. 3.4 Rotameter block. Typical arrangement of rotameters on an anaesthetic machine.

the mass of the bobbin is constant the force required to hold it is constant and so the pressure to keep it stationary (in terms of height) is constant. The orifice around the outside of the bobbin determines the resistance to flow. If flow is increased the pressure on the bobbin increases and it rises. The size of the orifice around the bobbin increases, reducing the resistance to flow and the pressure on the bobbin itself falls until it is maintaining the bobbin at a constant height again. Thus the height of the bobbin is related to the flow of gas in the tube, and a scale printed on the outside of the tube is used to read off the flow. In practice both the viscosity and density of the gas determine the position of the bobbin and the tube must be calibrated for each gas.

A number of factors may lead to inaccuracies:

- the tube is not kept vertical
- build-up of static electricity in the tube
- dirt in the tube

- build-up of back-pressure from any equipment placed down-stream of the vaporizers which restricts flow.

Gas flow can also be measured by sensing the pressure drop across a fixed resistance. Such a device is called a pneumotacho-graph.

SOLUBILITY

A gas placed with a liquid in a confined space will dissolve in that liquid. The amount dissolved in the liquid depends on the partial pressure of the gas in equilibrium with the liquid (Henry's Law). The quantity of gas that will dissolve in the liquid is also dependent on the solubility of the gas in the liquid and is described by the solubility coefficient. The partition coefficient describes how a substance distributes between two phases. This is defined as the ratio of the amount of the substance present in one phase compared with the amount present in a second phase, the two phases being of equal volume and in equilibrium. A solubility coefficient can only be applied to a gas and a liquid, but the partition coefficient can be applied to any two phases for example oil and water.

A liquid contains moving molecules held together by Van der Waal's forces. Some molecules have enough energy and hence velocity to escape from the surface of the liquid and form a vapour. As the temperature of the liquid is increased the number of molecules having sufficient energy to escape also increases. The total energy state of the remaining molecules is reduced and the liquid cools. At any temperature an equilibrium is reached where the number of molecules leaving the liquid phase is balanced by the number re-entering the liquid. At this point the vapour above the liquid is 'saturated'. When the temperature of the liquid is increased the pressure of the saturated vapour also increases and when the pressure of the saturated vapour is equal to the ambient pressure the liquid boils. Hence, the boiling point of a liquid is the temperature at which the saturated vapour pressure is equal to the ambient pressure.

EQUIPMENT

ANAESTHETIC MACHINE

At its most basic the anaesthetic machine is a device to deliver and regulate the flow of gas. Usually there is more than one gas and a typical machine provides supplies of oxygen, air and nitrous oxide. Gases are supplied either from pipelines at 400 kPa (4 bar) or from cylinders attached to the anaesthetic machine. Cylinder pressure is regulated by a reducing valve. Pressure gauges show the pressure in the pipelines and cylinders. The flow is controlled either by needle valves and variable orifice flowmeters (Rotameters) or electronically. Anaesthetic machines usually permit the placement of one or more vaporizers on a fitting which automatically diverts the fresh gas flow through the vaporizer. There is a mechanism to prevent more than one vaporizer being switched on at a time. In one system the displacement of a metal bar which protrudes from the vaporizer when it is turned on prevents any other vaporizer fitted to the same machine from being switched on (the Selectatec system). An oxygen flush control, which switches off automatically when released, supplies oxygen 100% at a flow rate of at least 35 L/min, bypassing the flowmeters and the vaporizers.

Anaesthetic machines contain a number of safety features to prevent a build up of pressure and to prevent the administration of a hypoxic mixture.

SAFETY FEATURES

- A safety valve on the machine prevents the pressure in the gas delivery system rising above 30–40 kPa.
- The gas flowmeters are linked either mechanically or pneumatically to prevent nitrous oxide being administered without oxygen.
- Whenever the machine is on, a minimum of 300 ml/min of oxygen is delivered.
- In the event of a failure of the oxygen supply an alarm will sound and the flow of nitrous oxide is terminated.

Other safety features on modern anaesthetic machines include:

- Non-interchangeable connectors on flexible pipelines to prevent incorrect connection.
- A system to prevent the placement of the wrong cylinder onto the yoke by which they attach to the anaesthetic machine (the pin-index system).
- Positioning the oxygen flowmeter downstream of the other flowmeters. Should any of the other flowmeters develop a leak,

this arrangement prevents a hypoxic mixture being administered as oxygen is the last gas to be added to the gas mixture.

Most anaesthetic machines have other apparatus attached to them such as a ventilator, monitoring equipment, scavenging equipment, suction equipment, electrical sockets, and lights. If the machine requires an electrical supply to operate, a battery backup will be present. Some newer designs are predominantly electronically controlled and may not have flowmeters or conventional vaporizers but rely on direct injection of volatile agents into the gas-flow. Their design is too complicated to consider further here.

SUPPLY OF GASES

Most anaesthetic rooms and operating theatres have a piped supply of the commonly used gases such as oxygen, air, and nitrous oxide as well as piped vacuum and scavenging of waste gases. Despite the presence of piped supplies, oxygen cylinders should always be available and attached to the anaesthetic machine in case of failure of the pipeline supply. Cylinders of other gases are often present but are not necessary. The supply of medical air and nitrous oxide to the pipelines is from a bulk cylinder store (called a manifold) within the hospital. Oxygen may be stored in large cylinders but in most medium and large hospitals a liquid oxygen store is used. This is a vacuum insulated flask kept away from the main hospital building. The gas pressure in the pipelines is maintained around 4 bar (400 kPa). A separate supply of medical air at 7 bar is also provided in orthopaedic theatres to power compressed air tools. All connections to piped gases are non-interchangeable.

Gas cylinders

Gas cylinders are made from molybdenum steel. They are pressure-checked every five years and a random sample of cylinders are cut apart to permit inspection for metal fatigue. The material between the neck of the cylinder and the valve melts at high temperature allowing the contents to escape if the cylinder is in a fire. The weight of the cylinder when empty is stamped on it so that the weight of its contents can be determined. Cylinders are colour coded to allow easy identification of the contents and are available in a range of sizes (Table 4.1).

The connection between the cylinder and anaesthetic machine is controlled by a pin-index system preventing incorrect fitting (see above). Gases supplied in cylinders include oxygen, medical air, nitrous oxide and carbon dioxide. There is no place for the routine

TABLE 4.1 Colour coding of gas cylinders used in anaesthesia

	Colour of body	Colour of shoulder	Pressure when full (100 kPa)
Oxygen	Black	White	137
Nitrous oxide	Blue	Blue	44
Carbon dioxide	Grey	Grey	50
Air	Grey	White/black quarters	137
Nitrous oxide/oxygen (Entonox)	Blue	White/blue quarters	137

use of carbon dioxide on anaesthetic machines and cylinders of this gas should only be attached when specifically needed and then removed immediately afterwards. However, carbon dioxide is frequently used elsewhere in the operating theatre to create a pneumo-peritoneum for laparoscopic surgery. Other gases which may be supplied in cylinders are helium/oxygen mixes and Entonox.

SCAVENGING

Anaesthetic gases which might otherwise be discharged from the anaesthetic circuit, the ventilator or anaesthetic machine into the room air in the operating theatre are removed by scavenging equipment and discharged into the external atmosphere. Although there is no evidence that occupational exposure to nitrous oxide leads to an increase in spontaneous abortion it is known to be toxic after long-term administration. The effects of long-term exposure to the volatile agents is unknown but, like nitrous oxide, is limited by the Control of Substances Hazardous to Health (COSHH) regulations in the UK. Production of waste gases can be limited by the use of low-flow systems and the prevention of leaks from the anaesthetic circuit and face-mask. Anaesthetic gases are collected from circuits and ventilators by scavenging systems. Most scavenging systems are active; a small negative pressure is generated to propel the gas into the outside atmosphere. A pressure-limiting device prevents a negative pressure being applied to the patient side of the breathing system.

> ⚠ **Care must be taken to prevent obstruction to scavenging systems which might otherwise create a resistance to expiration by the patient.**

VACUUM

Piped vacuum is available in most operating suites. To prevent fluids or solids entering the hospital pipework, filters and shut-off valves are present between the receptacle chamber and the vacuum supply. It is usually possible to regulate the vacuum.

ANAESTHETIC BREATHING SYSTEMS

These are often known as anaesthetic circuits and have previously been classified as open, semi-closed or closed (circle) systems. In an open systems the anaesthetic liquid is applied directly to material covering a face-mask such as the Schimmelbush mask. They are no longer in use in the UK.

The most useful classification is:

- non-rebreathing
- partial re-breathing
- rebreathing (circle).

Non-rebreathing systems contain a valve which prevents any contact between inspired and expired air. Although such a system may seem ideal it is wasteful of anaesthetic gases, requires a completely sealed system, may be complex with a number of valves which increase resistance to expiration and is to some extent futile because of mixing which must occur in the anatomical and equipment dead-space. However, such an arrangement may be seen in ventilators used on Intensive Care Units and portable ventilators used for resuscitation and transport of patients. If used in spontaneously breathing patients the supply of fresh gases must be at least equal to the peak-inspiratory flow rate. This is achieved either by the use of a reservoir bag, air-entrainment, or a demand valve attached to the gas supply system. One commonly used valve arrangement is the 'Ambu' valve which is used with a self-inflating bag and oxygen supply (Figure 4.1).

Breathing systems used for anaesthesia are either partial rebreathing or rebreathing (circle) systems. All anaesthetic breathing systems must have a fresh gas supply, a spill or expiratory valve to allow discharge of waste gas, and are made from wide-bore tubing so that there is as little resistance to gas flow as possible. During spontaneous ventilation the spill valve should be left in the fully open (anti-clockwise) position so that there is the least resistance to expiration. During controlled ventilation the valve may be set to open at higher pressures by use of a spring which presses against

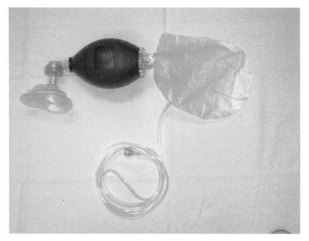

Fig. 4.1 Ambu non-rebreathing valve and reservoir bag.

the valve when the control is turned clockwise (Figures 4.2 and
4.3). This allows positive pressure to be generated in the breathing system and gas to pass into the patient's lungs. Spill valves are

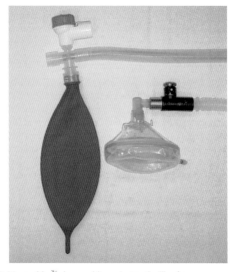

Fig. 4.2 Disposable and reuseable expiratory (spill) valves.

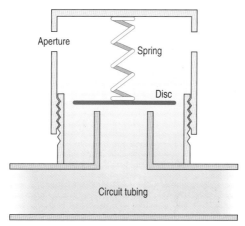

Fig. 4.3 Internal arrangement of expiratory valve.

designed to allow scavenging tubing to be attached. Most anaesthetic breathing systems are constructed of light-weight plastic and are usually labelled single-use only. The patient end is separated from the face-mask, tracheal tube or laryngeal mask airway by a filter that retains moisture derived from exhaled air and returns the moisture to inspired air. These filters also prevent passage of bacteria and viruses. At the time of writing their efficiency at preventing the passage of prions is unknown. Most manufacturers will approve the use of their breathing systems for more than one patient provided a filter is used.

PARTIAL REBREATHING SYSTEMS

In these systems inspired and expired air are deliberately allowed to mix. Rebreathing is controlled by altering the fresh gas flow rate. The degree of rebreathing will also be determined by apparatus dead space, leaks in the system and the patient's breathing pattern. These systems have been classified by Mapleson into five types (see Figure 4.4):

- Mapleson A (Magill attachment)
- Mapleson B
- Mapleson C (Water's circuit)
- Mapleson D (Bain coaxial system)
- Mapleson E (Ayre's T piece; Jackson-Rees modification – Mapleson F).

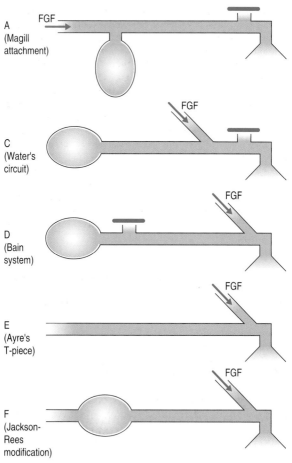

Fig. 4.4 Mapleson classification of partial rebreathing anaesthetic circuits with alternative names in brackets.

Mapleson A

This system is the most efficient during spontaneous ventilation. The first part of the exhaled gas (which contains little carbon dioxide as it was in the dead-space at the end of inspiration) fills the corrugated tubing. Once the corrugated tubing is full and the bag starts to distend the pressure in the system rises and the rest of the exhaled gas (the gas from the alveoli) is vented out of the system via the spill-valve. Thus the carbon dioxide-containing exhaled alveolar gas is discharged and carbon dioxide-free dead space gas is preserved and can be re-used without leading to rebreathing of carbon dioxide. As a consequence, the fresh gas flow can be set to alveolar volume (about 70–80% of minute volume). However, during controlled ventilation the Mapleson A system is much less efficient. During inspiration the pressure generated in the system by squeezing the bag causes a large proportion of the fresh gas in the tubing to be vented through the valve. The fresh gas flow must be at least three times alveolar minute volume to prevent rebreathing of carbon dioxide.

The original Mapleson A system is the Magill attachment in which the spill-valve is placed near to the patient connection. The Lack system places the spill valve away from the patient by using a second piece of corrugated tubing between the patient and the valve. The second tube may be parallel to the first or placed inside it. Both tubes must be of sufficient diameter to minimize resistance to flow. This modification does not significantly affect the mechanics of this system in use.

Mapleson B and C

These systems are very similar. The B is not used but the C system, often called the Water's circuit, is often seen. The original Water's circuit had a small canister of carbon dioxide absorbent in between

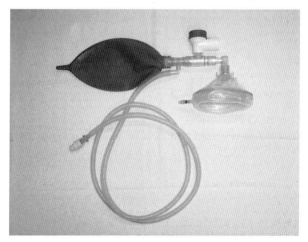

Fig. 4.5 Water's circuit often used during resuscitations and in recovery areas.

the reservoir bag and the patient. This is not used now, and the usual C circuit is shown in Figure 4.5. It is can be made small and light and is often used for resuscitation or to transfer patients. However, a high fresh gas flow is required to prevent rebreathing and a self-inflating bag and non-rebreathing valve are safer.

Mapleson D

The Mapleson D system is a modification of the T-piece. The fresh gas enters the circuit close to the patient and the spill valve and reservoir bag are distant. This system is inefficient during spontaneous ventilation when a fresh gas flow of twice the alveolar minute volume is required. During expiration the dead-space gas is preferentially lost through the spill-valve rather than alveolar gas which is retained in the system until the fresh gas flushes the alveolar gas out from the corrugated tubing. However, with controlled ventilation the Mapleson D system is more efficient than the Mapleson A system. The D system is available in a number of forms the commonest of which is the Bain coaxial system (Figure 4.6). Fresh gas is supplied through the inner narrower tubing. A simple 'bag-squeezer' type ventilator can be used with the Bain system when the ventilator connection replaces the bag. During controlled ventilation the spill valve is completely closed, excess gas being discharged through the ventilator.

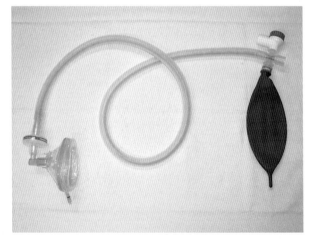

Fig. 4.6 Coaxial Bain circuit with fresh gas delivered through inner tubing and rebreathed and exhaled gas passing through outer tubing.

Mapleson E

This is also known as the Ayre's T-piece. Because there is no bag or spill valve there should be no resistance to expiration. It is used in paediatric anaesthesia when the Jackson Rees modification (Mapleson F) is used (Figure 4.7). In this system an open-ended bag is put on the end of the corrugated tubing. The bag increases the reservoir of fresh gas, enables visual inspection of breathing and may be used for controlled ventilation by occluding the open end of the bag and squeezing it. Like the Mapleson D system, the fresh gas flow should be at least twice the alveolar ventilation.

REBREATHING SYSTEMS

Breathing systems which allow rebreathing of all the exhaled gases can be safely used if the 'contaminants' of exhaled gas are removed. The main contaminant is carbon dioxide and this is usually removed by passing the gas through a container of soda lime. Soda lime contains:

- Calcium hydroxide
- Sodium hydroxide
- Potassium hydroxide
- Water
- Silica
- Indicator.

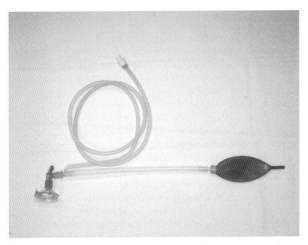

Fig. 4.7 Ayre's T-piece circuit used for small children and neonates.

Because soda lime is formed into granules and there are air spaces in between the granules, the surface area for reaction between the soda lime and carbon dioxide is huge. The major reaction is the combination of carbon dioxide and calcium hydroxide to form calcium carbonate and water. This is an exothermic reaction causing the soda lime to heat up. Silica prevents the granules breaking down into dust and the indicator changes colour when the soda lime is exhausted.

The main advantages of circle systems are the preservation of heat and moisture in the respiratory gases, and the cost reduction from use of less oxygen, nitrous oxide and volatile agent. In addition atmospheric pollution is reduced. Soda lime canisters vary in their capacity. A charge of 0.5 kg will maintain efficiency at clearing carbon dioxide for about 2–4 h. The larger 'jumbo' circles contain 1–2 kg of soda lime and last up to 8 h. Some circle systems have an internal volume of several litres, necessitating a prolonged period of flushing with gas mixture at the beginning of a case and also making them slower to respond to changes in the composition of the fresh gas flow. Circle systems (see Figures 4.8 and 4.9) usually consist of:

- a chamber containing the soda lime
- two one-way valves to ensure the gas travels in one direction only around the circle
- a spill valve
- a reservoir bag
- a fresh gas connection.

There is usually a switch to change from bag to ventilator. Some types allow the soda lime canister to be disconnected from the circuit during use so that the soda lime can be changed.

Circle systems require continuous monitoring of inspired gases, which is now mandated by recent guidelines. There are a number of problems with using low fresh-gas flow with circle systems. Vaporizers have altered output characteristics at low flows (less than 1 L/min). As the fresh gas flow is reduced the fraction of the oxygen supplied that is required for basal oxygen consumption rises towards 100%. However, after 30 min or so the uptake of nitrous oxide is minimal. Thus the expired gas may contain no oxygen, and only nitrous oxide and carbon dioxide are exhaled and the nitrous oxide concentration in the rebreathed gas may rise. Continuous gas analysis should warn of problems related to either of these issues. If the fresh gas flow is kept above 1 L/min these problems are not important clinically.

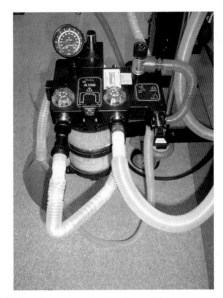

Fig. 4.8 Circle system with jumbo absorber canister.

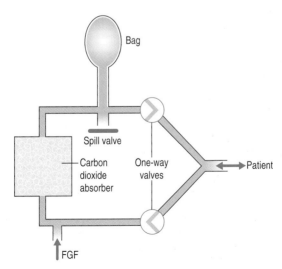

Fig. 4.9 Schematic drawing of components of a typical circle system.

VENTILATORS

Ventilators may be classified in a number of ways. Those present
on modern anaesthesia machines are in general electronically controlled and the mechanics of their operation are too complicated to
explain in detail. However, the basic principles of their operation
and control are considered below.

MINUTE VOLUME DIVIDER

A type of ventilator rarely seen now, the 'minute volume divider'
simply divides the fresh gas flow into a series of breaths of
predetermined tidal volume. The many iterations of the Manley
ventilator are mostly simple minute volume dividers which use only
the supply pressure of the fresh gas to power them.

'BAG-SQUEEZER'

Most modern anaesthetic machines have a built-in ventilator
operating via a circle system. The basic design is that of a 'bag-
squeezer' (Figure 4.10). The ventilator mimics manual compression of the reservoir bag. The connection to the circle is separate
from the reservoir bag but the bellows in the ventilator can be
considered as another bag. This 'bag' is squeezed by gas contained in the plastic container and pressing on the outside of the
bag. Thus these ventilators are also called 'bag-in-a-bottle' ventilators. The bag or bellows separates the anaesthetic gas in the
circle system from the driving gas of the ventilator. The characteristics of the respiratory cycle produced by these ventilators are
controlled electronically. Usually the tidal volume and the respiratory rate are set by the user. Other factors which may be set are
the ratio of the duration inspiration to expiration, the inspiratory
flow rate, and the amount of positive end-expiratory pressure.
Some ventilators allow a number of modes of ventilation. The
usual mode used is intermittent mandatory volume (sometimes
called 'volume control'). A set number of breaths of a set tidal
volume are delivered. Other modes may compensate for spontaneous breaths the patient may initiate (used on ICU) or provide

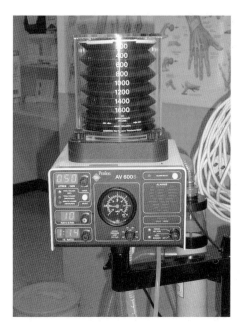

Fig. 4.10 Typical bag-squeezer ventilator.

pressure-controlled ventilation. In this mode the respiratory rate, the length of inspiration and the inspiratory pressure are set. The tidal volume will then depend on the compliance of the patient's chest wall and lungs. All these modes are monitored by sensors which detect respiratory pressure and volumes. Alarms are provided, the most important of which is the 'low pressure' alarm. If there is a disconnection between the ventilator and the patient, the pressure fails to rise above a minimum value during the respiratory cycle and the alarm sounds. Some ventilators automatically compensate for changes in the fresh gas flow rate and for changes in compliance of the patient or the circuit. Unfortunately there is little standardization on the design of these ventilators and the user new to a particular ventilator must ensure he/she is familiar with its use before the anaesthetic is started.

AIRWAY DEVICES

TRACHEAL TUBES

Tracheal tubes are designed for single use only and are manufactured from inert plastic. Tubes for adult anaesthesia are provided with a cuff which is inflated to form a seal between the tube and the wall of the trachea. Tubes are available in a range of sizes but for adults an 8.0 mm internal diameter tube is usually used for women and a 9.0 mm tube for men. Straight from the packet, new tubes are too long and are usually cut to 22 cm length for women and 23 cm for men before use. This places the connection between the anaesthetic circuit and the tube near the patient's mouth. Too long a tube may bend and kink as the tube heats up to body temperature and becomes softer. A tube cut too long may also be inserted too far and increase the risk of endobronchial intubation.

There are a number of specialized tubes (Figure 4.11) such as those which are reinforced to resist kinking and used when the head is manipulated during surgery (such as in neurosurgery or maxillo-facial surgery), narrow tubes to permit laryngoscopic examination of the vocal cords (microlaryngeal tubes), tubes with a preformed shape to direct the tube away from the mouth (either upwards or downwards) used in ENT and maxillo-facial surgery, and tubes resistant to laser light.

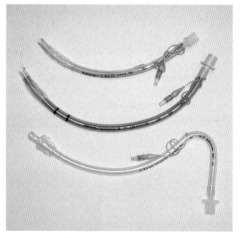

Fig. 4.11 A selection of tracheal tubes – standard oral tube, reinforced tube, nasal tube (top to bottom).

LARYNGEAL MASK AIRWAY

This device (see Figure 4.12) sits in the laryngopharynx so that its cuff surrounds the laryngeal inlet. It does not seal inside the tracheal lumen and so does not isolate the trachea or protect the airway against aspiration of stomach contents. The laryngeal mask airway was designed to be used in spontaneously breathing patients; however, the seal is reasonably airtight and some anaesthetists use them as a means to provide positive pressure ventilation of the lungs. The pressure in the cuff should not be allowed to exceed 60 cm H_2O. The device is inserted with the cuff deflated and is well tolerated in deeply anaesthetized patients without the use of muscle relaxants. Different sizes are available depending on the weight of the patient (Table 4.2). Standard laryngeal mask airways are sterilized after each use. Single-use laryngeal mask airways and other similar supraglottic airway devices are now available.

FACE-MASK

Black rubber face-masks have been used for many years but have now been replaced with disposable, clear plastic face-masks. An appropriate size is chosen for the patient that provides an airtight seal around the mouth and nose.

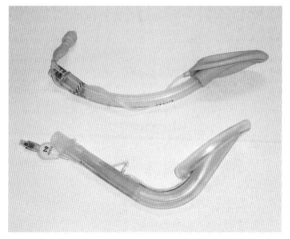

Fig. 4.12 Reusable (top) and single-use (disposable) (bottom) laryngeal mask airways.

TABLE 4.2 Recommended maximum inflation volume for the re-useable laryngeal mask airway

Patient weight (kg)	LMA size	Recommended maximum volume of air in cuff (ml)
<5	1	4
5–10	1½	7
10–20	2	10
20–30	2½	14
30–50	3	20
50–70	4	30
70–100	5	40

AIRWAYS

Most oral airways are of the Guedel type (Figure 4.13). These are sized by choosing an airway the same length as the distance from the angle of the jaw to the corner of the mouth. Nasal airways are also available and are better tolerated during recovery or in semi-conscious patients (Figure 4.14).

LARYNGOSCOPES

A number of different laryngoscope designs are available. The commonest is the curved or Macintosh laryngoscope (Figure 4.15). The

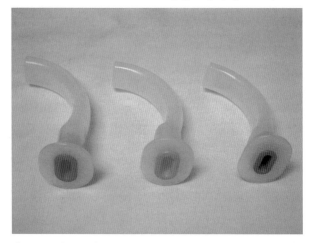

Fig. 4.13 Selection of oral Guedel airways.

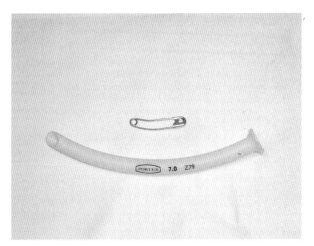

Fig. 4.14 Nasal airway and retaining safety pin.

adult blade is available in two sizes – standard and long. The laryngoscope is held in the operator's left hand and the tip is designed to sit in the vallecula (the space between the back of the tongue and the base of the epiglottis). The laryngoscope is lifted along the long axis

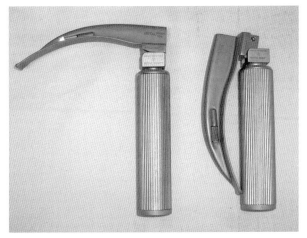

Fig. 4.15 Macintosh laryngoscope.

of the handle to lift the tongue and epiglottis up and allow visualization of the laryngeal inlet and vocal cords.

> ⚠ **Care must be taken not to lever the laryngoscope handle backwards and cause the blade to rock against the upper teeth.**

MONITORING

One of the most important advances in anaesthesia in the last 15–20 years has been the improvement in monitoring of even the most basic physiological functions. Only a few years ago anaesthesia monitoring consisted of an ECG, blood pressure (probably measured by a manual oscillotonometer) and the anaesthetist's finger on a peripheral pulse. Today, all locations where anaesthesia is administered should have basic monitoring available. The minimum requirements have been described by the Association of Anaesthetists of Great Britain and Ireland (AAGBI) (Table 5.1).

TABLE 5.1 Minimum monitoring standards

Induction of anaesthesia	Pulse oximeter Non-invasive blood pressure Electrocardiography Capnography
Maintenance of anaesthesia	Pulse oximeter Non-invasive blood pressure Electrocardiography Capnography Vapour analyser
Recovery	Pulse oximeter Non-invasive blood pressure

In addition a nerve stimulator and a means of measuring the patient's temperature must be available

Adapted from: Recommendations for standards of monitoring during anaesthesia and recovery 3. London: Association of Anaesthetists of Great Britain and Ireland, 2000.

In addition to the monitoring described in the table, other modalities are commonly used. Direct measurement of arterial and central blood pressure is common. Transoesophageal echocardiography, measurements of pulmonary artery pressure, cerebral blood flow and oxygenation and cerebral electrical function such as EEG are used in specialist situations.

Modern monitoring equipment is provided with alarms. The limits outside which the alarm is triggered may be factory set, determined by the user or set themselves within a predetermined percentage of the initial reading (for example ± 20% of the first blood pressure reading).

> ⚠ **Alarms systems can only be as good as the accuracy of the monitor, the correct setting of the alarm limits, the attention given to alarm warnings and the use of appropriate action after an alarm is triggered.**

CARDIOVASCULAR SYSTEM

ELECTROCARDIOGRAM (ECG)

The ECG provides information on the cardiac rate, the rhythm and semi-quantitative information on the presence of ischaemia. The usual configuration is to record standard lead II using three electrodes. However, if the right arm lead (red) is placed over the manubrium, the left arm lead (yellow) over the apex and the indifferent electrode (black) on the left shoulder the CM5 lead, which is more sensitive at detecting ischaemia, is created. For many arrhythmias and changes in the PQRS pattern a full 12-lead ECG is required to correctly diagnose the abnormality.

PERIPHERAL BLOOD HAEMOGLOBIN OXYGEN SATURATION (PULSE OXIMETRY)

A probe is placed over an extremity such as a digit or earlobe. The transmission of light produced by two light-emitting diodes (LED) through the extremity is recorded by a photodetector. The transmission is altered by the light-absorbing characteristics of haemoglobin which alters with the relative proportions of oxy-haemoglobin and deoxyhaemoglobin. By using two different frequencies (one from each LED) an algorithm determines the ratio of these two haemoglobin states. The saturation of haemoglobin in the arterial blood is determined by removing the contribution of the non-pulsatile (tissue and venous) components.

Because of the shape of the haemoglobin dissociation curve (see Figure 1.2), the peripheral blood oxygen saturation may remain in the 'normal' range despite a marked fall in partial pressure of oxygen. Once the steep part of the dissociation curve is reached small falls in partial pressure then produce more dramatic changes in saturation.

Pulse oximeters may fail to function correctly:

- if carboxyhaemoglobin or methaemoglobin are present
- with poor peripheral perfusion
- with excessive ambient light
- with movement artefact
- with use of diathermy.

⚠️ **A probe placed on an extremity should be moved every 4 hours. The slight heating effect and the use of spring clips can result in skin ischaemia.**

BLOOD PRESSURE

Arterial blood pressure can be measured by a traditional sphygmomanometer, by oscillotonometry, an automated version of the oscillotonometer or by direct pressure measurement.

Traditional sphygmomanometry using auscultation of Korotkoff sounds is impracticable during anaesthesia and surgery. Oscillotonometry uses the pulsation in the artery palpable just distal to an inflated cuff as that cuff is slowly deflated below arterial systolic pressure. The pulsations are due to opening and closing of the artery vessel walls when the occluding pressure is between systolic and diastolic pressure. Above systolic pressure no distal pulsation is detected and when the occluding pressure is below the diastolic pressure the vessel remains permanently open. Originally a double-cuff was used but modern automated machines use a single-cuff technique. This method is inaccurate at low pressures (<60 mmHg) and may underestimate the true pressure at high systolic pressures. These machines may also have difficulty in obtaining a reading if the arm is being moved or if the cuff is incorrectly placed on the arm. Repeated frequent use may cause skin petechiae and nerve compression. The cycle time of most monitors can be set by the user and every 2.5 or 3 minutes is usually satisfactory.

> ⚠️ **Accurate measurement requires use of a cuff of adequate width, which should be at least 1.2 times the diameter of the limb.**

The blood pressure may be measured directly by an arterial cannula placed in a peripheral artery such as the radial artery at the wrist or the dorsalis pedis artery in the foot. To measure central venous pressure the venous system is usually cannulated at the great vessels in the neck (either the internal jugular or subclavian vein) and the tip advanced so that it lies within the thorax. Alternatively a 'long line' may be passed up the veins of the arm from the antecubital fossa and into the great veins of the thorax.

Indications for direct measurement of arterial pressure:

- major surgery likely to produce heavy blood loss
- use of vasoactive drugs or techniques likely to lead to swings in blood pressure
- major co-morbidity
- need for frequent blood samples (for example for blood gas analysis).

Complications of arterial cannulation:

- haemorrhage
- damage to the artery
- thrombosis and occlusion (rarely leads to ischaemia)
- infection.

Indications for central venous pressure measurement:

- monitoring of cardiac 'filling' pressures if major blood loss expected
- use of vasoactive drugs that must be given into a great vein
- administration of hyperosmolar solutions (e.g. parenteral feed).

Complications of central venous cannulation:

- venous injury
- arterial injury
- thoracic duct injury
- pneumothorax and haemothorax
- pericardial tamponade
- arrhythmias
- infection – local and systemic
- embolus
- thrombosis.

The cannula is connected to a transducer by fluid-filled, low-volume, stiff-walled tubing. The transducer is 'zeroed' at a reference level (usually the height of the left ventricle for arterial pressure recording and the right atrium for CVP measurements). Careful attention to prevent air bubbles or kinks in the cannula or the tubing which might dampen the system is essential.

RESPIRATORY SYSTEM

The respiratory system can be monitored by:

- measuring the airway pressure during the respiratory cycle
- spirometry
- measuring the oxygen concentration in the fresh gas flow
- measurement of gases in the anaesthetic circuit near to the point of connection with the patient.

AIRWAY PRESSURE

Most modern anaesthetic machines and their associated ventilators continuously measure and display airway pressure. Such a device may

TABLE 5.2 Causes of an increase in airway pressure

Cause	Example
Reduction in chest wall compliance	A reduction in the degree of muscle paralysis
Reduction in lung compliance	Pneumothorax
Increase in airway resistance	Kinked circuit Kinked tracheal tube Bronchospasm

form part of a disconnection alarm (if the circuit becomes detached from the patient the airway pressure fails to reach a predetermined level during each respiratory cycle and an alarm is triggered). Causes of an increase in airway pressure are given in Table 5.2.

SPIROMETRY

Volume and flow can be measured in the anaesthesia circuit by a respirometer or a pneumotachograph. These should be sited in the expiratory limb of the circuit as near to the patient as possible. Flow–volume loops can be displayed and with simultaneous measurement of pressure, compliance can be calculated.

OXYGEN MEASUREMENT

Continuous measurement of oxygen in the fresh gas flow is an integral part of anaesthesia monitoring and also forms part of the anaesthesia machine checklist recommended by AAGBI.

There are a number of techniques to measure oxygen content continuously:

- fuel (galvanic) cell
- polarographic or Clark electrode
- paramagnetic analyser
- mass spectroscopy[*]
- Raman spectroscopy.[*]

The most common technique is the fuel cell in which an electric current, produced by a chemical reaction, is dependent on the partial pressure of oxygen in contact with the electrodes. As fuel cells respond to the partial pressure of oxygen and not the concentration, they will be affected if they are placed in a high pressure part of the circuit. They need to be calibrated regularly and have a limited lifespan. With a suitable alarm they can be used

------

[*]may also be used to measure anaesthetic gases.

to prevent administration of a hypoxic mixture. They can also be used to confirm that pure (100%) oxygen is being delivered by the anaesthetic machine during the machine check.

GASES IN THE ANAESTHETIC CIRCUIT

The concentration of other gases including carbon dioxide, nitrous oxide and the commonly used anaesthetic vapours is usually determined by infra-red spectroscopy. These gases are measured continuously in expired air. Continuous measurement of carbon dioxide is known as capnography. When displayed graphically the capnograph may indicate changes in the respiratory pattern such as evidence of expiratory obstruction due to chronic airways disease, or partial obstruction of the anaesthetic circuit or airway (Figure 5.1).

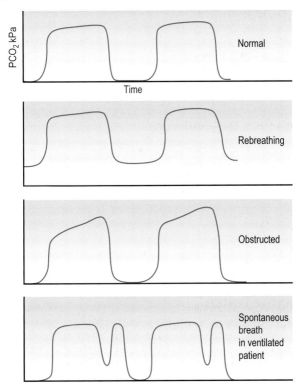

Fig. 5.1 Normal capnograph trace and examples of abnormal traces.

Confirmation of the correct placement of a tracheal tube is provided by detection of carbon dioxide in the expired air. A sudden decrease in expired carbon dioxide may indicate an increase in dead-space due to an obstruction in the pulmonary circulation after an embolus.

MONITORING OF THE NEUROMUSCULAR JUNCTION

Assessment of neuromuscular blockade assists in determining the onset of block, depth of block during surgery, suitability for reversal of blockade and the achievement of recovery from blockade.

The muscle response to nerve stimulation is assessed either by visual, tactile or mechanical means. A peripheral nerve is stimulated and the supplied muscle observed. Common sites are the ulnar nerve proximal to the wrist causing stimulation of the adductor pollicis (see Figure 5.3), the lateral popliteal nerve near the head of the fibula with assessment of the peroneal muscles, or the facial nerve just anterior to the ear producing movement of the orbicularis orbis musculature. Visual estimation of the response to stimulation is the least reliable technique. Tactile response is most frequently used clinically. Mechanical methods may be used quantitatively but are generally reserved for research use and include mechanomyography (force transducer), electromyography (summation of muscle action potentials) and accelerography (acceleration). Skin surface electrodes are used. The delivered current should be about 20% more than is required to stimulate all the fibres in the nerve and ensure maximum muscle response. Usually a current of 50 mA for 0.2 ms is sufficient.

A number of patterns of stimulation are used:

- single-twitch
- tetany
- train-of-four
- double burst stimulation
- post-tetanic count.

SINGLE TWITCH

The single twitch may be repeated every 10 seconds and a reduction in twitch height relative to a control twitch obtained prior to neuromuscular blockade indicates the degree of receptor blockade. However, at least 75% of receptors must be blocked before any reduction in twitch height is observed.

TETANY

Tetanic stimulation at 50 or 100 Hz will detect fade (a gradual
reduction in the contraction during continuous stimulation) due to
non-depolarizing blockade. Tetanic stimulation can also be used to
produce facilitation in the post-tetanic count test. This test is useful
to determine profound blockade due to non-depolarizing agents.
A tetanic stimulation at 50 Hz is applied for 5 seconds and after a
3 second gap, a single twitch is applied every 1 second. The tetanic
stimulation produes facilitation so a twitch will appear even if
there is profound blockade. The number of twitches which can be
counted after the tetanic stimulation can be used as a measure of
the block. A count of 10 occurs at about the stage of recovery from
deep blockade when the first twitch of the train-of-four response
reappears. A count of less than 10 indicates profound blockade.

TRAIN-OF-FOUR

The train-of-four pattern is four stimuli applied over 2 seconds at a
rate of 2 Hz (Figures 5.2 and 5.3). With small degrees of block due
to a non-depolarizing agent, fade is seen during the four twitches.
The ratio of the fourth to the first twitch height is known as the
train-of-four ratio. As block deepens the fourth, then the third,

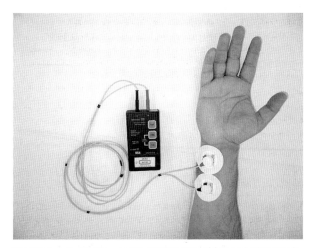

Fig. 5.2 Typical stimulator used to generate train-of-four and other stimuli
of peripheral nerves.

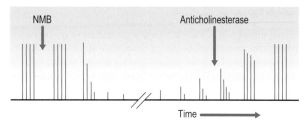

Fig. 5.3 Changes in train-of-four trace after administration of non-depolarizing neuromuscular block agent, as the block starts to wear off, and after administration of an anti-cholinesterase.

then the second and eventually the first twitch response disappear and on recovery the twitch responses reappear in the reverse order. Adequate block for surgical exposure of abdomen is found when only the first twitch is present. Generally, reversal of block with an anti-cholinesterase should only be attempted when at least two twitches are present. Adequate reversal has occurred when all four twitches are present and the train-of-four ratio is 0.7 or greater. The train-of-four stimulus can be repeated every 12 seconds.

DOUBLE BURST STIMULATION

For double burst stimulation two short bursts (three impulses each) of tetanic (50 Hz) stimulation are given separated by 0.75 second. The fade of the second burst relative to the first may be easier to detect than fade during train-of-four stimulation but indicates the same degree of block as the train-of-four ratio.

TEMPERATURE

Temperature measurement is recommended for all patients. It is essential during any procedure where temperature is likely to fall significantly. General anaesthesia inhibits the body's ability to maintain temperature. In addition a number of factors may contribute to loss of heat including open body cavities, use of cool and dry gases, use of room temperature fluids for intravenous replacement and for lavage, and exposure of large areas of body surface. Rapid increases in temperature may indicate a hypermetabolic state such as malignant hyperthermia. Temperature probes may be inserted into the nasopharynx, oesophagus or rectum. The probes contain a thermistor whose resistance varies with temperature.

DEPTH OF ANAESTHESIA

Depth of anaesthesia is currently only monitored in specialist areas such as the use of electroencephalography and evoked responses during spinal and carotid artery surgery and also for research purposes. New techniques which use processed EEGs combined with frontalis EMGs such as the bispectral index monitor are not yet used widely. There is evidence that their use may be associated with a reduced risk of awareness in some situations.

PREOPERATIVE ASSESSMENT

PREOPERATIVE ASSESSMENT AND PLANNING

The preoperative assessment should be used to establish a patient–doctor relationship. It is important to use appropriate history taking and examination to assess the surgical and medical health of the patient, in particular the severity of any systemic illnesses and the risk of perioperative morbidity. For elective cases the opportunity should be taken to optimize the patient's medical condition to minimize the risk of perioperative morbidity. The patient should be given a brief and appropriate explanation of procedures and risks, have any questions answered and (hopefully) their fears and anxiety reduced; the aim should be to give the correct information in a reassuring manner. If necessary, preoperative medication can be prescribed.

SUGGESTED SCHEME FOR PREOPERATIVE ASSESSMENT

It is important to have a scheme of preoperative assessment so that all important aspects are covered (Table 6.1).

TABLE 6.1 Checklist for pre-anaesthetic assessment

History:

Co-existing illnesses
Medications
Exercise tolerance
Problems with previous anaesthetics, or family history of problems
Allergies

Examination:

Weight
Blood pressure
Dental health
Assessment for difficult airway including Mallampatti classification
Back/limbs if regional blocks planned
Other systems as appropriate

Other information:

Results of relevant investigations
Expert opinion, referrals
ASA classification
Information given to patient
Nil by mouth status
Premedication
Prophylaxis
Information to HDU/ICU if indicated

HISTORY

The history and review of the medical notes should aim to get information on the following topics:

Surgical condition

Information about the surgical condition and proposed operation is important to get an insight into the extent and duration of the proposed surgery, the expected fluid and blood loss, the type of incision and the need for intraoperative and postoperative analgesia. If the operation is an emergency (or urgent), the patient might have a full stomach. An assessment of the fluid status and the response to resuscitation up to that time is also required.

Co-existing medical illness

A systemic approach should be followed in making an assessment of co-existing medical illnesses. It is important to evaluate if the illness is under control and if there has been any recent change in the severity or treatment. It is also important to ascertain whether a speciality referral or further investigations are required for full evaluation. The speciality referrals are not to determine 'fitness' for anaesthesia, but to assess the severity of illness and to ascertain if anything else can be done to optimize the condition.

Ischaemic heart disease, asthma, chronic obstructive pulmonary disease, hypertension and diabetes are commonly seen in surgical patients and are associated with significant perioperative risks (Table 6.2). The relevance of these factors is discussed further in Chapter 7.

Exercise tolerance

This is assessed by determining the patient's maximum level of activity, and can be used to predict overall outcome. It is affected by age, but gives a good indication of cardio-respiratory reserve. The assessment may be difficult if activity is limited by arthritis. Patients with moderate limitation of exercise (has to stop because of breathlessness or angina after a 100-yard brisk walk or climbing two flights of stairs) may require further investigation and assessment of current therapy. Those with severe limitation of exercise (breathlessness on minimal activity such as walking a few yards; unable to climb one flight of stairs without stopping) will require invasive monitoring perioperatively and HDU/ICU admission postoperatively.

TABLE 6.2 Some common medical conditions and associated risks

Upper respiratory tract infection	Bronchospasm at induction, intubation, or extubation Laryngeal spasm at induction, intubation, or extubation Spread of infection causing pneumonia
Asthma	Severe bronchospasm during induction, intubation or extubation Mucous plugging Postoperative pneumonia
Ischaemic heart disease	Worsening ischaemia and ventricular dysfunction Arrhythmias Perioperative myocardial infarction Complications are more likely in cases of recent infarction (<3 months) and unstable angina
Hypertension	Labile blood pressure perioperatively Arrhythmias Myocardial ischaemia Stroke Left ventricular failure
Diabetes	Hypoglycaemia/hyperglycaemia Autonomic dysfunction – arrhythmias, hypotension Silent myocardial ischaemia/infarction Gastro-oesophageal reflux
Arthritis	Difficulty in opening mouth for laryngoscopy and intubation Difficult positioning Unstable cervical spine

Medications

Knowledge of the precise dose, schedule and type of medication(s) is important. Particularly important are drugs acting on the:

- cardiovascular system (antihypertensives, antianginals, antiarrhythmics)
- clotting system (anticoagulants)
- endocrine systems (antidiabetic agents, steroids)
- bronchomotor tone
- nervous system (antidepressants, anticonvulsants).

Some medications have to be discontinued (anticoagulants) or modified in dose (insulin). However, most drugs should be continued up to the time of operation (in particular antihypertensives, antianginal drugs), and resumed as soon as possible afterwards.

Anaesthesia-related problems

Any problems with previous anaesthetics should be ascertained from the old records (as the patient may not be aware of them) and by direct questioning. The following aspects will influence the perioperative management:

- any problems with airway management – in particular previous difficult laryngoscopy and intubation
- response to pain control measures and any untoward effects of opioids
- postoperative nausea and vomiting and response to treatment
- prolonged recovery
- unexpected HDU/ICU admission
- other unexpected complications or drug reactions such as malignant hyperthermia, succinylcholine apnoea and anaphylaxis.

Allergies/drug reactions

True allergic or hypersensitivity reactions are less common than non-allergic, unpleasant side-effects. The distinction is usually made by asking specific questions. Skin manifestations (urticaria, rash), bronchospasm, cardiovascular collapse and/or angioneurotic oedema should be taken as true allergic reaction unless proven otherwise. Apart from anaesthetic agents, allergies to antibiotics, adhesive tapes, latex, sprays and particular types of food are important to note; these would influence the choice of anaesthetic technique (Table 6.3). Latex allergy has become more common (or perhaps more commonly recognized) recently. A history of allergic reactions after contact with rubber products including condoms, urinary catheters or surgical gloves warns of this allergy. There are

TABLE 6.3 Allergies and anaesthetic implications

Allergy	Implications
Antibiotics	Choice of antibiotics for prophylaxis
Shellfish, sea food	Cross-reactions with iv contrast agent and protamine
Egg yolk, soyabean	Possible cross-reaction with propofol
Ester local anaesthetics	Choice of agent
Latex	Latex free gloves, i.v. sets, catheters, tracheal tubes, monitoring devices and other equipment
Adhesive tapes	Use hypoallergic variety

also cross-reactions to certain fruits such as kiwi fruit. Contact dermatitis after exposure to latex is common and is not necessarily associated with anaphylaxis to latex. Most products (with the notable exception of surgical and non-sterile gloves) are latex-free.

Social history

Details of smoking, alcohol intake and substance abuse are important. In smokers, the presence of a productive cough may indicate the need for further evaluation and treatment. Stopping smoking even for up to 12 h significantly reduces the amount of carboxyhaemoglobin in blood and improves oxygen delivery to tissues. The beneficial effects on airway reactivity and secretions are not seen (in the form of reduced pulmonary complications) until 4 weeks after stopping. Acute alcohol intoxication lowers the requirement for anaesthetics and may lead to hypothermia and hypoglycaemia. Withdrawal from alcohol can cause agitation, confusion, hypertension, palpitation and seizures. Stimulant abuse predisposes to arrhythmias and convulsions. Recent stimulant use may increase the requirment for anaesthetic agents (increase in MAC). Opioid abuse increases the doses of these agents required perioperatively.

PHYSICAL EXAMINATION

All patients should be weighed.

Head, neck and airway

Examination of the airway is mandatory in all patients undergoing anaesthesia. Any obvious deformities, the degree of mouth opening, the range of cervical spine movement, tracheal deviation, lesions in the oral cavity or in the neck have important implications (Table 6.4). The size of the mandible should be assessed by measuring thyromental distance (distance from the lower border of the mandible to the thyroid notch with the neck fully extended). If this distance is less than 6.5 cm, laryngoscopy is more likely to be difficult. Another test for the predicted ease or difficulty of laryngoscopy and tracheal intubation is the Mallampati classification (Table 6.5). The assessment is made with the patient sitting upright and the head in neutral position. The patient is asked to first open his/her mouth as widely as possible, protrude the tongue fully and then say 'aah'. The visible structures in the oral cavity should be noted. Classes 3 and 4 are more likely to be associated with difficult laryngoscopy. However, these tests are neither fully sensitive or specific.

TABLE 6.4 Conditions associated with difficulty in airway management

Nose:	
Deviated septum	Difficult insertion of nasotracheal tube, bleeding
Polyps	Same as above
Mouth:	
Facial scars and contractures	Restricted mouth opening
Macroglossia	Difficulty in visualizing larynx on laryngoscopy
Prominent incisors	Same as above and prone to damage
Poor dentition	Prone to damage or loss
Caps and crowns	Protect from damage
Mandible:	
Receding or short mandible	Difficulty in visualizing larynx on laryngoscopy
TMJ problems	Difficulty in opening mouth, symptoms worsen after mandibular manipulation for airway management
Neck:	
Burn contractures	Difficulty in visualizing larynx on laryngoscopy
Tracheostomy scars	Tracheal tube of smaller diameter
Short thick neck	Difficulty in laryngoscopy
Goitre/other swellings	Deviated or compressed upper airway
Cellulitis	Deviated, compressed or swollen upper airway
Restricted movement	Difficult laryngoscopy, potential for trauma
Rheumatoid arthritis	Evidence of atlanto-axial subluxation, or neurological symptoms on neck movement – careful fixation of head after induction and during intubation

Chest and precordium

Physical examination of heart and lungs should be carried out according to the clinical condition. In all patients the lung fields should be auscultated for evidence of normal respiration.

TABLE 6.5 Mallampati classification

Class 1: Visible pharyngeal pillars, soft palate and uvula
Class 2: Uvula masked by tongue; pharyngeal pillars and soft palate still visible
Class 3: Only soft palate visible; pharyngeal pillars and uvula completely masked
Class 4: Only hard palate visible; pharyngeal pillars, soft palate and uvula completely masked

Abdomen

Where appropriate abdominal distension should be noted as it signifies an increased risk of regurgitation and pulmonary aspiration.

Neurology

The conscious state, if altered, should be noted. Also any evidence of existing neurological problems (for example hemiparesis, or neuropathies) should be noted; this may be useful if neurological symptoms are reported after general or regional anaesthesia.

Back (spine)

Infection of the skin is a contraindication for spinal or epidural injection. Any spinal deformity would also predict difficulty in performing these procedures and potential for neurological damage (hence a relative contraindication).

Extremities

The upper limbs should be examined for suitable sites of venous cannulation. If local blocks are planned, anatomical landmarks should be examined and any evidence of skin infection should be noted as these may contraindicate placement of local anaesthetic blocks.

INVESTIGATIONS

Routine preoperative laboratory investigations are now discouraged; the tests should be tailored to the individual patient. The National Institute for Clinical Excellence has produced guidelines and most hospitals have their own version of these. The following should be taken as a guide.

Haemoglobin

Healthy patients undergoing elective surgery with expected blood loss <10% of total blood volume do not require estimation of haemoglobin.

Estimation is required in:

- Neonates <6 months
- Women >50 years

- Men >65 years of age
- Sickle cell disease or trait
- Malignancy
- Haematological disorder
- Preoperative blood loss
- Trauma
- Malnutrition
- Other systemic illnesses and ASA 3 or above (see below).

Urea and electrolytes

Not indicated in healthy patients undergoing elective surgery.
Indications include:

- Patients >65 years
- Renal disease
- Diabetes
- Hypertension
- Ischaemic or vascular heart disease
- Liver disease
- Patients receiving digoxin, diuretics, steroids, ACE inhibitors and antiarrhythmic agents.

Rapid correction of electrolyte abnormality in an otherwise stable patient can cause problems, such as central pontine demyelination while correcting hyponatraemia, and arrhythmias while correcting hypokalaemia. If possible, the operation should be delayed and any abnormality corrected slowly (over 2–3 days for hyponatraemia).

Clotting studies

Indicated in:

- Known bleeding disorder or coagulopathy
- Anticoagulants therapy
- Recent blood transfusion replacing >20% of total blood volume
- Recent infusion of colloids or other plasma substitutes replacing >20% of total blood volume (total blood volume is roughly 70–80 ml/kg body weight)
- Unexplained bruising
- Unexplained blood loss and/or reduced haemoglobin
- Hypersplenism
- Liver disorder
- Renal failure.

Electrocardiogram

This is indicated in:

- Men >40
- Women >50
- Cardiovascular disease
- Renal disease
- Diabetes
- Electrolyte imbalance
- Known arrhythmias
- Patients on antihypertensive, antiarrhythmic or antianginal agents.

A recent (within 3 months) change in the ECG should be considered significant and warrants further investigation.

Chest X-ray

Indicated in:

- Chest disease
- Exercise-limiting cardiovascular disease
- Long standing smoker with symptoms or signs of chest disease
- Malignancy.

In most of these conditions a recent (within the previous 3 months) CXR is satisfactory unless there has been a change in symptoms or signs.

Other investigations

Other investigations may be required for full assessment of the severity of disease, effectiveness of treatment, and whether or not the patient is in optimum medical condition and the risks involved. These investigations may include:

- lung function tests
- arterial blood gases (lung disease with limited exercise tolerance)
- echocardiography (heart disease with indication of limited function)
- exercise ECG (coronary artery disease with angina)
- liver enzymes (alcoholism, liver disease)
- blood glucose (diabetes)
- endocrine functions (hypo/hyperthyroidism).

Some investigations are also required to establish a baseline preoperative level for comparison with intra- and postoperative changes (for example arterial blood gases).

ASSESSMENT OF RISK OF ANAESTHESIA

Assessment of risk is important to:

- document the complexity of medical conditions
- obtain informed consent
- arrange appropriate level of help
- make necessary arrangements for perioperative care (invasive monitoring, HDU/ICU care).

The overall complexity of clinical condition can be assessed by American Society of Anesthesiologists (ASA) physical status classification (Table 6.6). ASA class 4 or more and most ASA class 3 do not qualify for day-case surgery, and often require more intensive monitoring and high dependency postoperative care. Class 1 and 5 are self-explanatory. The differentiation between classes 2 and 3, and classes 3 and 4 is not precise. However, typical examples of classes 2, 3 and 4 are:

- Class 2 – treated hypertension without complications
- Class 3 – coronary artery disease with angina during moderate exertion
- Class 4 – recent myocardial infarction with heart failure.

Of the deaths reported in the 1999 NCEPOD report, 84% were patients with an ASA class >3. Various other scoring systems have been described to assess risks in patients with cardiac, respiratory or systemic illnesses and these have been described in the relevant sections of this book.

INFORMATION TO THE PATIENT AND CONSENT

Patients may have fear, anxiety or concerns related to surgery and anaesthesia, and in the information and explanation you should

TABLE 6.6 ASA Classification	
Class 1	A healthy patient
Class 2	Mild systemic disease
Class 3	Severe systemic disease that may limit activity but is not incapacitating
Class 4	Severe systemic disease which is incapacitating and is a constant threat to life
Class 5	Moribund, not expected to live for 24 hours with or without operation

If the procedure is performed as an emergency, an 'e' is added to the ASA class *not* comment on questions specifically related to surgery (i.e. surgical prognosis, scars, disfigurement, restriction on lifestyle). Anaesthesia related anxieties include death, awareness and/or pain during surgery, not waking up, postoperative pain, loss of control and nausea and vomiting. Try to explore these anxieties and reassure the patient:

- Offer an unhurried explanation.
- Be realistic about the risks, but in a reassuring manner. Patients have a right to know about common risks (those with an incidence over 1%, Table 6.7), and risks which may cause significant or permanent harm.
- Explain what will be done to avoid or minimize the risks.
- Describe what the patient should expect (cannulations, monitoring devices) before induction of anaesthesia and in recovery.
- Discuss the choice of anaesthetic technique (GA or regional) in view of the patient's preferences and previous experiences.
- Discuss the alternative if the proposed plan doesn't work (i.e. general anaesthesia if a regional block fails).

All discussion should be carried out in simple, non-jargon, layperson terms. The amount of information given to the patient will depend on his/her willingness to know and pre-existing knowledge.

TABLE 6.7 Common complications

Regional anaesthesia

Headache (subarachnoid block)
Local bleeding
Nerve injury
Partial effect

General anaesthesia

Sore throat
Hoarse voice
Dental injury
Postoperative nausea and vomiting
Other complications specific to pre-existing illness (i.e. bronchospasm in asthmatics, cardiac dysfunction in known cardiac disease)

Vascular cannulation

Discomfort
Haematoma
Thrombosis
Pain
Infection

PREOPERATIVE PREPARATION OF THE PATIENT

Generally, for elective surgery:

- Adults should not eat solids for 6 hours before an operation. They can have a light breakfast in the morning when the operation is scheduled for the afternoon.
- Children and infants can have solids and/or milk up to 6 hours before operation.
- All patients can have clear fluids for up to 2 hours before surgery.
- Babies are allowed to breast feed or be given formula feed up to 4 hours before surgery.

The reason for preoperative fasting is to minimize the volume of the stomach contents and the associated risk of regurgitation and pulmonary aspiration after induction of anaesthesia. Despite adequate fasting, some patients may still be at the risk of regurgitation and pulmonary aspiration; these patients have either a slow gastric emptying or decreased lower oesophageal sphincter tone or both (Tables 6.8, 6.9). Antacid prophylaxis should be prescribed in these patients and tracheal intubation should be performed using the rapid-sequence method; these patients are not suitable for laryngeal mask airway. Patients presenting for emergency surgery are often considered as having a full stomach even if they have been starved for these times. Clearly those with an acute abdomen will have gastric stasis. However, stasis can also be induced by anxiety, pain and opioid analgesics.

PREMEDICATION

This is rarely used in adults except when there are specific indications. However it may be necessary:

- to reduce excessive patient anxiety
- provide pain relief (if necessary) for movement, positioning and procedures (cannulations, regional analgesia) before induction of anaesthesia
- for specific indications, e.g. anatacid prophylaxis, glyceryl trinitrate patch.

TABLE 6.8 Factors associated with decreased lower oesophageal sphincter tone

Obesity
Pregnancy (after the first trimester)
Hiatus hernia
Gastro-oesophageal reflux disease
Abdominal distension
Drugs:
- atropine, glycopyrrolate
- opioids
- volatile anaesthetics

TABLE 6.9 Factors decreasing the rate of gastric emptying

Physiological

Acid
High protein content food
Pregnancy

Pathophysiological

Anxiety
Trauma
Surgery
Shock
Pain
Diabetes

Drugs

Opioids
Anticholinergics
Tricyclic antidepressants

Children are often given sedative premedication and a topical local anaesthetic cream is applied to the skin at the site of intended venous cannulation.

Benzodiazepines, opioids and anticholinergics are the traditional anxiolytics.

Benzodiazepines

Temazepam 10–20 mg given orally 1–2 hours before surgery produces sedation and amnesia without prolonged sedation after operation. Diazepam 5–10 mg given orally 1–2 hours before surgery produces sedation, but this may be prolonged after surgery. In the anaesthetic room, intravenous midazolam 1–3 mg provides amnesia and sedation.

Opioids

The main indication for opioids is to relieve pain preoperatively (fractures, acute abdomen). Morphine 5–10 mg i.m. 60–90 min before surgery is sufficient. Opioids are often combined with an anti-emetic (for example cyclizine 50 mg).

Anticholinergics

The main indication is to reduce oral secretions in adults and to prevent bradycardia during induction in children. Glycopyrrolate can be used in the dose of 0.2–0.4 mg i.v. for adults and 10–20 µg/kg for children.

Prophylaxis for Aspiration Pneumonitis

At the induction of anaesthesia the cough reflex is lost and any regurgitant from the stomach can be aspirated into the trachea. The severity of any resulting aspiration pneumonitis depends on the acidity (pH) of the stomach contents and their volume. Patients who are particularly at risk include pregnant women, those with a hiatus hernia, gastro-oesophageal reflux, difficult airway, ileus, and obesity (also see Tables 6.8 and 6.9). Drugs can be used to minimize gastric secretions and the volume of gastric contents.

Histamine (H₂) antagonists and proton-pump inhibitors

Ranitidine 150–300 mg orally or 50–100 mg i.v./i.m. reduces the acidity and volume of gastric contents. Proton-pump inhibitors such as omeprazole are an alternative.

Antacids

Non-particulate antacids such as sodium citrate 30–60 ml can be given immediately before induction of anaesthesia.

Prokinetics

Metoclopramide, a dopamine antagonist, can be used to enhance gastric emptying with simultaneous increase in the tone of lower oesophageal sphincter. There is little evidence that such agents significantly reduce the risk of regurgitation.

PRE-EXISTING DISEASE

Many patients presenting for anaesthesia suffer from unrelated illnesses such as hypertension or chronic obstructive pulmonary disease (COPD). These illnesses affect the function of the body and may influence the choice of anaesthetic agents, the anaesthetic technique and the outcome. In addition, drug treatment may also interact with anaesthetic agents. Perioperative management of the elderly, obese and patients with diabetes is described in Chapter 13 and in the Action Plans (Chapter 19).

CARDIOVASCULAR DISEASE

The aims in patients suffering with cardiovascular disease are:

● Optimize preoperative state to reduce the risk from factors known to influence outcome (see Table 7.1).

TABLE 7.1 Primary and secondary risk factors for perioperative cardiac morbidity

Risk factors	Risks
Primary risk factors	
Congestive heart failure	Sudden death, arrhythmias, prolonged postoperative ICU admission
Unstable angina	Perioperative MI, heart failure, arrhythmias
Recent MI	High risk of re-infarction if the operation is performed within 3 months of previous MI. This risk is reduced to <2% if the operation is delayed for 6 months
Uncontrolled hypertension	Arrhythmias, congestive heart failure, stroke
Arrhythmia (ventricular arrhythmias and supraventricular tachycardia indicate underlying myocardial disease)	Congestive heart failure, and myocardial ischaemia
Secondary risk factors	
Diabetes mellitus	Increased mortality
Smoking	Increased risk of ischaemic heart disease
Obesity	Increased incidence of perioperative myocardial ischaemia
Age	Increased incidence of perioperative myocardial ischaemia
Vascular disease	Increased incidence of perioperative myocardial infarction

- Apply appropriate perioperative monitoring and support to minimize further deterioration in cardiac function.
- Use an appropriate anaesthetic technique to maintain adequate circulation and prevent secondary organ damage during anaesthesia and surgery.

It is important to understand the factors that can affect myocardial oxygen supply and demand (Chapter 1). These are modified by the effects of disease and of anaesthesia.

PREOPERATIVE ASSESSMENT

Take a full history and determine the patient's exercise tolerance (a useful indicator of the severity of illness). Ensure that major reversible risk factors such as cardiac failure, myocardial ischaemia, angina, arrhythmias and hypertension are well controlled. Recent changes (within the previous 3 months) in the severity of any of these conditions should be investigated prior to elective surgery. Note the dose, frequency and any side-effects of concurrent therapy. Table 7 2 shows the cardiovascular drugs that are commonly used and their implications for anaesthesia. Assess the need for optimization of medications.

For a full and detailed evaluation of cardiac function, a 12-lead ECG, exercise tolerance test (in patients with suspected ischaemic heart disease), echocardiography (to give an indication of myocardial function, chamber size and valvular function), and cardiac catheterization (rarely indicated as part of an anaesthetic assessment alone) may be required. A summary of the indicators of good or impaired left ventricular function is given in Table 7.3. Various scoring systems have been used to assess the risk of a perioperative major cardiac event. One such scoring system is described in Table 7.4. None of the currently available scoring systems have been shown to be completely reliable.

ANAESTHESIA

There is no evidence that regional or general anaesthesia is inherently safer. The underlying principle is to maintain the myocardial oxygen demand–supply balance. To achieve that:

- avoid sympathetic stimulation
- avoid myocardial depression
- avoid swings in blood pressure

TABLE 7.2 Concurrent medications

Drugs	Implications during anaesthesia
Beta adrenoreceptor antagonists (beta-blockers)	Continue perioperatively Preoperative cessation can cause rebound hypertension, angina or myocardial infarction. Incremental glycopyrrolate or atropine can be given to treat perioperative bradycardia
Calcium channel antagonists	Continue perioperatively Verapamil can predispose to AV block if combined with halothane
ACE inhibitors	Can cause hyperkalaemia Can precipitate severe hypotension in hypovolaemic patients at induction of anaesthesia Can predispose to renal failure
Digoxin	Assess dosage in the elderly and in patients with renal disease Measure serum potassium and avoid hypokalaemia
Diuretics	Measure serum potassium perioperatively
Oral anticoagulants	Avoid spinal/epidural anaesthesia unless warfarin fully reversed Stop warfarin at least 48 hours preoperatively Use heparin infusion in high risk patients (e.g. metal heart valves) and stop just prior to surgery, restart as soon as possible after surgery INR should be <1.5 times control Use fresh frozen plasma if unexpected or severe haemorrhage Restart warfarin on first postoperative day after minor surgery After major surgery start heparin infusion on first postoperative day and continue until warfarin is restarted
Aspirin/clopidogrel	Stop 1–2 weeks before surgery Can increase oozing from wound Regional blocks should only be performed by experienced anaesthetists High index of suspicion for postoperative haematoma formation in patients with epidural blockade

TABLE 7.3 Indicators of good or impaired left ventricular function

Good function	Impaired function
Good exercise tolerance	Limited exercise tolerance
Essential hypertension	History of MI, heart failure
Ejection fraction more than 0.5	Ejection fraction less than 0.4
LVEDP less than 12 mmHg	LVEDP more than 18 mmHg
Good global contractility on echocardiography	Areas of dyskinesia (abnormal movement) or akinesia on echocardiography

TABLE 7.4 Modified Goldman's Index of cardiac risk in patients undergoing non-cardiac surgery

Risk factor	Points
Third heart sound indicating heart failure	11
MI in preceding six months	10
Rhythm other than sinus or premature atrial contractions	7
More than five ventricular ectopic beats per minute	7
Abdominal, thoracic or aortic surgery	3
Age more than 70 years	5
Aortic stenosis	3
Emergency operation	4
Poor condition as indicated by any one of PaO_2 less than 8 kPa, $PaCO_2$ more than 6.5 kPa, potassium less than 3 mmol/litre, HCO_3 less than 20 mmol/litre, urea more than 7.5 mmol/litre, creatinine more than 270 μmol/litre, SGOT abnormal, chronic liver disease	3
Total	**53**

Incidence of major cardiac complications:
0–5 points; up to 3%
6–12 points; up to 10%
13–25 points; up to 30%
26–53 points; up to 75%
Adapted from Goldman L et al (1977) N Eng J Med 197:848.

- maintain heart rate and blood pressure within 20% of the baseline value
- safe analgesia without cardiovascular depression.

Induction of general anaesthesia

- Etomidate is the least cardiovascular depressant of the currently available intravenous induction agents. However it has a number of unpleasant side-effects (see Chapter 2). Thiopental or propofol should be given slowly to avoid a sudden drop in blood pressure. Laryngoscopy and tracheal intubation are often associated with tachycardia and hypertension and a short-acting opioid (alfentanil or fentanyl) should be given along with the intravenous induction agent to attenuate the cardiovascular response. Muscle relaxants such as atracurium, vecuronium and rocuronium have minimal cardiovascular effects. In patients with moderate or severe cardiovascular disease an arterial line placed prior to induction may help guide the induction and the treatment of any cardiovascular sequelae.

Maintenance of anaesthesia

If general anaesthesia is used, a balanced technique is safest. Pay meticulous attention to fluid and electrolyte balance. Monitoring should be continued into the postoperative period.

Postoperative period

Unstable patients should be admitted to an HDU or ICU ward. Regional analgesia and nerve blocks provide excellent analgesia without the risk of respiratory depression. But these techniques may be associated with sympathetic block which can lead to postoperative hypotension and therefore patients must be monitored carefully. Usual medication should be restarted as soon as possible and intravenous substitutes should be used if oral medication is not possible.

SPECIFIC CONDITIONS

Hypertension

Elective surgery should not be undertaken if hypertension is poorly controlled (for example a diastolic pressure >105 mmHg). Hypertensive patients undergoing anaesthesia are likely to have episodes of hypotension or hypertension during the perioperative period. Hypotension is particularly likely after induction of anaesthesia and after subarachnoid block. Induction of anaesthesia should be slow and the dose of intravenous agent carefully titrated to prevent cardiovascular depression. Treatment with beta-adreno-receptor antagonists (beta-blockers) and reduced left ventricular compliance in hypertensive patients impairs the physiological response to hypovolaemia or blood loss and invasive monitoring such as central venous pressure monitoring is indicated for major procedures. Pain is the main cause of postoperative hypertension.

Ischaemic heart disease

Postoperative myocardial infarction has an associated mortality of 40–60%. Elective surgery should be postponed for at least three and probably six months after a myocardial infarction. Poorly controlled or unstable angina increases the risk of perioperative MI and should be fully investigated and treated before surgery. In emergency situations, low dose aspirin (150 mg/day) and systemic heparinization may decrease the risk. Anaemia should be corrected. Patients on calcium channel antagonists and/or ACE inhibitors can develop severe hypotension, especially with volatile anaesthetic agents. Normocapnia should be maintained during anaesthesia. Hypercapnia can lead to arrhythmias while hypocapnia can cause coronary artery vasoconstriction and a shift of the oxyhaemoglobin dissociation curve to the left leading to decreased oxygen delivery to the myocardium.

Heart failure

Anaesthesia and surgery are contraindicated with recent or uncontrolled heart failure. Although many anaesthetic agents cause vasodilatation and reduced afterload, which helps patients with heart failure, many also reduce contractility. Patients with controlled heart failure are often receiving chronic diuretic therapy that makes them prone to hypotension during further vasodilatation. Electrolyte disturbances should be corrected prior to anaesthesia.

Arrythmias

Sinus bradycardia from beta-adrenoreceptor blockade is common and not harmful. Atrial or ventricular premature contractions are usually benign. Underlying causes such as ischaemic heart disease or electrolyte disturbance should be assessed. Atrial fibrillation is increasingly common as age advances. Causes such as thyrotoxicosis and mitral stenosis should be excluded. If atrial fibrillation is chronic and cannot be converted back to sinus rhythm, the ventricular rate should be controlled prior to anaesthesia. In the elderly digoxin levels should be measured. Other arrhythmias such as supraventricular and ventricular tachycardias, frequent premature contractions associated with cardiovascular compromise and heart block warrant cardiological referral prior to anaesthesia.

Patient with a permanent pacemaker

If not checked within the previous six months, a permanent pacemaker should be reviewed. Diathermy should be used only if absolutely necessary. If possible use bipolar rather than unipolar diathermy. If unipolar diathermy must be used, place the indifferent electrode on the same side of the body as the operating side and as far away from the pacemaker as possible. Watch the ECG for signs of pacemaker inhibition.

> ⚠️ A permanent magnet placed over a demand pacemaker may convert it to a fixed-rate device. However, modern pacemakers have sophisticated programming systems used after insertion which may be reset by a permanent magnet. Advice should be sought from a cardiological centre – preferably the one where the patient is routinely monitored.

RESPIRATORY DISEASE

The main concerns in patients with significant respiratory disease are maintenance of adequate gas exchange perioperatively and the prevention of postoperative respiratory failure. It is important to consider the effects of anaesthesia on respiratory function as well as the impact of respiratory disease on the conduct of anaesthesia.

EFFECT OF ANAESTHESIA ON RESPIRATORY FUNCTION

General anaesthesia, the supine position and abdominal surgery all decrease the functional residual capacity, promoting airway closure and atelectasis during tidal breathing. This increases ventilation/ perfusion (V/Q) mismatch and causes hypoxaemia. Upper airway instrumentation, use of dry anaesthetic gases and anaesthesia-associated depression of ciliary activity lead to damaged airway epithelium, thickened secretions and atelectasis and predispose to infections. Intermittent positive-pressure ventilation can cause further V/Q mismatch. Vital capacity may be reduced postoperatively, especially after abdominal and thoracic surgery and impaired coughing leads to retention of secretions. Additionally, anaesthetic agents and opioids impair the cough reflex and the respiratory response to hypoxaemia and hypercarbia. Other factors that can contribute to poor respiratory function perioperatively are in Table 7.5. The risk factors for perioperative morbidity and mortality are listed in Table 7.6.

PREOPERATIVE ASSESSMENT

Respiratory function and reserve should be assessed by:

- Determination of exercise tolerance (an indicator of the severity of illness).
- Investigation of chronic cough, wheeze, dyspnoea, or infection.
- Smoking history.
- Recent chest X-ray, lung function tests and arterial blood gases. A chest X-ray is not required for simple asthma, or stable mild chronic obstructive pulmonary disease. Arterial blood gases provide a useful baseline prior to major surgery.
- ECG.

Preoperative optimization of lung function
A number of factors in respiratory illness can be improved preoperatively:

- Stopping smoking for > 24 hours significantly reduces carboxy-haemoglobin in the blood; stopping for >4 weeks improves ciliary function and reduces airway secretions.

TABLE 7.5 Patient factors impairing respiratory function during anaesthesia

Advanced age
Pre-existing lung disease
Chest wall/spinal deformity
Smoking:
- decreased ciliary activity
- increased sputum production
- increased carboxyhaemoglobin

Obesity
Inadequate control of bronchospasm

TABLE 7.6 Risk factors for perioperative morbidity and mortality in patients with respiratory disease

Right heart failure (cor pulmonale)
Orthopnoea
Patient requiring home-oxygen therapy
Limited exercise tolerance
FEV_1 <1 L
VC <50% of predicted
Hypoxaemia and/or hypercarbia
Abdominal/thoracic surgery

- Bacterial analysis of sputum and treatment of chest infection with antibiotics.
- Chest physiotherapy including breathing exercises, coughing, and incentive spirometry.
- Management of bronchospasm with bronchodilators.
- Inhaled/systemic steroids in patients with reversible airways disease.
- Control of pulmonary hypertension with long-term oxygen therapy.

ANAESTHESIA

Patients undergoing spinal or epidural anaesthesia alone may not tolerate lying supine during long operations. Persistent coughing can also be a problem. A combined general anaesthetic and regional technique may be preferable. Aim for adequate ventilation without hypoxaemia or hypercapnia, and early extubation and return of spontaneous respiratory function with an adequate cough at the end of surgery. Postoperative respiratory depression (for example from opioids) increases complications; use regional techniques for analgesia if possible.

High-risk patients should be admitted to an HDU or ICU facility postoperatively. The risk of atelectasis, sputum retention and pneumonia can be reduced by good pain relief without sedation or cough suppression, the use of humidified oxygen therapy and appropriate physiotherapy.

SPECIFIC CONDITIONS

Asthma

The risks of intraoperative bronchospasm mean that asthma must be controlled prior to anaesthesia/surgery. Clinical evaluation by history and examination should ascertain the severity and degree of control of the condition. Elective surgery should be postponed during any episode of inadequate control. Signs of poor control include increased wheeze, chest infection, cough and nocturnal dyspnoea. A history of previous use of NSAIDs should be taken. A small number of asthmatics are sensitive to these agents. Preoperative lung function testing is required in severe asthmatics, prior to major surgery, and those with repeated hospitalizations or ICU admission. Bronchospasm can by worsened intraoperatively by:

- poor preoperative control
- tracheal instrumentation
- light levels of anaesthesia
- extubation during light anaesthesia
- anaesthetic agents known to release histamine.

For well-controlled asthmatics, general or regional anaesthesia may be used. For more severe asthma, use regional anaesthesia if possible. If a general anaesthetic is necessary avoid agents which are known to release histamine such as thiopental, morphine and atracurium. Avoid tracheal intubation if possible. In patients at high risk of developing bronchospasm or prior to emergency operations in poorly controlled asthmatics, consider nebulized salbutamol (5 mg in normal saline 2–5 ml) 1 hour preoperatively, and hydrocortisone 1–2 mg/kg. Remember that volatile anaesthetics dilate bronchi.

Chronic obstructive pulmonary disease

Patients with COPD have an increased risk of postoperative chest infections, respiratory failure, right heart failure and arrhythmias.

TABLE 7.7 Factors predisposing to complications in patients with COPD

Obesity
Advanced age
Dyspnoea on mild exertion
Orthopnoea
$FEV_1/FVC < 60\%$
Atrial fibrillation and right heart failure
Recurrent chest infections
Previous ICU admissions for respiratory failure
Hypoxaemia on breathing air or carbon dioxide retention
Hypoxic respiratory drive
Home oxygen therapy
Upper abdominal/thoracic surgery

> **TABLE 7.8 Optimization of lung and cardiac function in patients with COPD**
>
> **Optimization of lung function**
>
> Regular inhaled bronchodilators (e.g. salbutamol, ipratropium)
> Inhaled or systemic steroids
> Antibiotics
> Physiotherapy and sputum clearance
> Oxygen therapy
>
> **Optimization of cardiac function**
>
> Oxygen
> Digoxin for right heart failure or atrial fibrillation
> Diuretic

Clinical evaluation should look for risk factors associated with these complications (see Table 7.7). Routine surgery should be postponed during an acute exacerbation (usually caused by a chest infection). Preoperative preparation should include stopping smoking for as long as possible, optimization of lung function (see Table 7.8) and treatment of right heart failure if present.

The anaesthetic technique is similar to that used for asthmatics. In addition maintain spontaneous ventilation if possible to prevent problems with stopping IPPV; avoid hypoxaemia or hypercarbia resulting from inadequate breathing; avoid nitrous oxide in the presence of bullae; and arrange admission to HDU/ICU after major procedures.

CONDUCT OF ANAESTHESIA

PRINCIPLES OF SAFE ANAESTHETIC PRACTICE

Anaesthesia is a relatively high-risk speciality; 70% of accidents in anaesthesia can be attributed to human error on a background of system failure. Therefore, a thorough understanding of the principles underlying safe practice in anaesthesia is of paramount importance. These principles should be incorporated into everyday practice right from the beginning of training in anaesthesia.

RISKS OF ANAESTHESIA

The mortality rate directly attributed to anaesthesia is estimated to be 1 in 10,000. Whilst the mortality remains relatively low in anaesthesia, the complication rates are much higher. Many complications are related to preventable causes:

- hypovolaemia
- hypoxia
- hypotension
- airway problems
- drug errors
- aspiration
- inadequate emergency management.

Various factors have been recognized which contribute to the development of critical incidents, leading to complications. These factors can be related to theatre environment, equipment, patient, surgeon or anaesthetist and are summarized in Table 8.1. Table 8.2 summarizes the important causes of death, cerebral damage and other complications related to anaesthesia. Many of the complications during anaesthesia and the factors which contribute to them are potentially preventable. Table 8.3 lists some of the other complications.

ESSENTIALS OF SAFE PRACTICE

Proper preoperative preparation is important (see Table 8.4). It is essential to have a clear anaesthetic plan and a back-up plan in case of problems. Trainees must ensure that they have communicated with all members of the team, including nursing staff, theatre staff, surgeons, ICU and senior anaesthetists. It is important that the anaesthetist realizes the limitations and human factors involved with surgeons, theatre staff and other members of the team. Do not attempt a procedure for the first time without direct or close supervision. Senior help should be sought in good time and

TABLE 8.1 Factors contributing to critical incidents

Factor	
Environment	• Ambient conditions
Equipment	• Design flaw • User error • Malfunction • Failure to report problems preoperatively
Patient	• Underlying disease • Inadequate risk assessment • Poor communication
Surgeon	• Failure to assess seriousness of pre-existing medical illness • Failure to appreciate the possible complications related to anaesthesia and surgery • Lack of communication with anaesthetists and other members of staff with regard to the extent of surgery and implications postoperatively
Anaesthetist	• Lack of skill • Lack of vigilance (human factors) • Failure to communicate with members of staff, surgeons, emergency team and ICU/HDU with regard to the risk assessment and management of patients

TABLE 8.2 Important causes of death or cerebral damage related to anaesthesia

Failure to establish airway or misplaced tracheal tube
Pulmonary aspiration
Hypoxia
Accidental pneumothorax
Drug errors
Miscalculation of dosage
Mismatched blood transfusion
Misuse of apparatus

TABLE 8.3 Other complications related to anaesthesia

Dental damage
Peripheral nerve damage
Awareness
Spinal cord damage
Injuries due to falls or burns
Allergic reactions

TABLE 8.4 Checklist before induction of anaesthesia

Make sure:
- that you have the correct patient for the correct procedure
- the surgical side is marked and is confirmed by the patient
- the patient has consented for the procedure
- the patient has followed the nil-by-mouth regime
- you are fully aware of any relevant co-morbidity and predicted anaesthetic complications
- senior help is available if needed
- you have plans for postoperative care (e.g. HDU or AICU)
- you have checked the anaesthetic machine
- you have all the necessary equipment
- you have drawn all the necessary drugs into labelled syringes

---

preferably before a case where you suspect there may be a potential complication. Avoid stressful conditions such as pressure to rush cases in order to meet the demand of the workload, an uncomfortable ambient temperature, long hours and fatigue, hunger and illness.

Preoperative and postoperative visits are essential components to assure a good quality of care to all patients undergoing anaesthesia. Document communication with other members of staff and medical teams or surgical teams and the steps taken to optimize patients' conditions. Documentation of the process of anaesthesia in terms of preoperative assessment, risk assessment, induction, maintenance, and immediate postoperative period should be clear, detailed and legible. Follow local and national standards and guidelines with regard to monitoring, adverse events, resuscitation and pain management.

OPERATING THEATRE ENVIRONMENT

Many aspects of the operating theatre environment will be new to a trainee embarking on a career in anaesthesia. For most anaesthetists, much of their working life is spent in the operating theatre and it is important to become familiar with its environment from the beginning. It is also important to familiarize yourself with the measures which are in place to ensure the safety of patients and staff. Most operating theatres have policies with regard to sterile zones. It is important to understand what precautions are expected from members of staff moving in and out of these areas.

ANAESTHETIC ROOM

In Britain, most hospitals have anaesthetic rooms where the majority of patients are anaesthetized before being taken into the operating room. These rooms are equipped with monitoring equipment, anaesthetic equipment, drugs, intravenous cannulae, intravenous fluids and various aids for tracheal intubation and maintenance of the airway. The advantages of having anaesthetic rooms are reduced patient anxiety and time saving – connecting the patient to monitors, establishing intravenous lines, etc., while the theatre is being prepared. The disadvantages are duplication of anaesthesia equipment and the temporary disconnection from the anaesthetic machine and monitoring during the transfer from the anaesthetic room into the operating theatre.

Seriously ill and unstable patients (for example emergency caesarean section, massive bleeding) are taken directly into theatre and anaesthetized there.

OPERATING THEATRE

These are designed around a centrally situated operating table. The outlets for piped gases, electrical sockets, anaesthetic machines and monitors should be located at the head-end of the table. The control of temperature, humidity and ventilation are important aspects of theatre environment. The temperature should range between 20 and 22°C with relative humidity between 50 and 60%. Higher temperatures may be required during operations involving extensive burns (associated with increased temperature loss) and neonates or infants. Air conditioning regulates the temperature and humidity and air is exchanged several times per hour. For certain procedures when the ambient lighting has to be dimmed (for example laparoscopic procedures) a light should be provided on the anaesthetic machine.

HAZARDS

These include electrical hazards, exposure to vapours, chemicals, radiation and infection. In addition, psychological stress results from working in a closed environment and constant demands on alertness and interaction with other members of staff. Various epidemiological surveys and studies have raised awareness with

> ⚠ **Hand washing between cases and proper use and appropriate disposal of needles and infected material is vital in minimizing the risks to staff and patients.**

TABLE 8.5 Factors affecting the environmental levels of volatile anaesthetic agents

Scavenging
Air conditioning and ventilation
Use of closed circuits and low flow
Keeping the flow of nitrous oxide switched off when the anaesthetic machine is not in use
Regular maintenance of equipment

TABLE 8.6 Precautions against spread of infection in the operating theatre environment

1. Wash hands between patient contact or on contamination with blood or body fluid
2. Wear gloves when touching mucous membranes or if there is the possibility of exposure to blood or body secretions
3. Dispose and handle all sharps (such as needles, scalpel blades) carefully, avoiding needle-stick injuries to yourself as well as to other members of the staff
4. In case of needle-stick injury, encourage bleeding and wash thoroughly and then follow local hospital procedures
5. Cover all your cuts, abrasions and open skin lesions with a waterproof dressing

regard to the potential hazards resulting from long-term exposure to anaesthetic vapours particularly nitrous oxide. However, providing exposure to anaesthetic vapours is minimized by effective scavenging there is no evidence of harmful consequences. Measures which help to keep these levels low are given in Table 8.5.

Precautions to minimize the risks of infection are given in Table 8.6.

CONDUCT OF GENERAL ANAESTHESIA

The primary aim of general anaesthesia is to provide:

- unconsciousness (hypnosis)
- analgesia
- optimal surgical conditions.

PREPARATION

INTRAVENOUS ACCESS

The patient may arrive in theatre with an intravenous cannula in situ; if so inject 5–10 ml of normal saline to ensure that the cannula is patent and that the saline does not extravasate or cause pain on injection. The size and number of intravenous cannulae required will vary according to the proposed procedure, the anticipated blood loss, and preoperative state of the patient. At least one 16 G cannula should be placed in an adult patient in whom blood loss is expected or who may require large volumes of fluid for other reasons (e.g. before spinal anaesthesia). In fit, healthy patients undergoing minor procedures a smaller cannula (18 G or 20 G) is satisfactory. A description of the technique to insert a cannula is given in Table 9.1.

ESTABLISH MONITORING

Standard monitoring should be in place before anaesthesia is induced (see Chapter 5). A nerve stimulator (whenever a muscle relaxant is used) and a means of measuring temperature should also be available. Invasive monitoring may be placed prior to

---

TABLE 9.1 Technique of intravenous cannulation

1. Ensure good light
2. Infiltrate the dermis with local anaesthetic (0.2 to 0.5 ml of 2% lidocaine) if a cannula larger than 18 gauge is to be inserted
3. For children apply EMLA at least 60 min before cannula insertion
4. The dorsum of the hand is the most convenient; avoid the antecubital fossa or veins close to arteries
5. Use gravity, warmth, a tourniquet and/or tapping on the overlying skin to dilate the vein prior to cannulation; the vein should not only be visible but it should also feel 'full' before the cannulation is attempted
6. Use a normal saline flush to ensure patency and correct placement before injecting any drugs
7. Secure in place with tape or sterile dressing.

induction, if the patient is haemodynamically unstable or if instability is expected during the induction of anaesthesia.

PRE-INDUCTION MEDICATIONS

Premedication given on the ward before leaving for the operating theatre is now infrequently used. Some specific indications are:

- a very anxious patient
- child (often topical local anaesthesia such as EMLA)
- requirement for an antisialogue, for example prior to awake fibreoptic intubation
- an H_2 antagonist or a proton pump inhibitor in a patient at risk of reflux
- cardiac anaesthesia (to prevent tachycardia and hypertension).

In the anaesthetic room benzodiazepines or short-acting opioids are frequently given as part of the anaesthetic induction technique (co-induction). Patients who are at increased risk of reflux and aspiration of gastric contents may be given sodium citrate (30 ml of a 0.3 M solution) just prior to induction of anaesthesia.

INDUCTION OF ANAESTHESIA

For induction the patient should lie on a tiltable trolley or bed. Most patients are preoxygenated to provide some degree of reserve during periods of apnoea (see later). Anaesthesia is induced using an intravenous or sometimes an inhalational technique. If laryngoscopy and tracheal intubation are necessary a muscle relaxant is given. However, it is advisable to test the ability to ventilate the lungs with face-mask ventilation before administering the relaxant. The exception to this rule is rapid-sequence induction. During laryngoscopy and tracheal intubation, it is important to ensure an adequate depth of anaesthesia by starting the maintenance drug(s) before the induction drugs have worn off.

STAGES OF ANAESTHESIA

The classical stages of anaesthesia and their signs were first described by Guedel, and were based on patients who were premedicated with morphine and were breathing ether (diethyl ether) in air for the induction of anaesthesia. The signs associated with anaesthesia using modern agents follow a similar course, but the divisions between stages are less distinctive:

Stage 1: Amnesia: this begins with the induction of anaesthesia and continues to loss of consciousness.

Stage 2: Stage of excitement: this is characterized by uninhibited excitation and potentially harmful responses to noxious stimuli including vomiting, laryngospasm, hypertension, tachycardia and uncontrolled movement. The pupils are often dilated, gaze may be divergent, respiration is irregular and breath holding is common.

Stage 3: Surgical anaesthesia: this is the target depth for anaesthesia. The gaze is central, pupils are constricted or normal sized and respiration is regular. Anaesthesia is considered sufficient when painful stimulation does not elicit any hypertension, tachycardia or movement.

Stage 4: Stage of impending respiratory and circulatory failure: this stage is marked by shallow or absent respiration, dilated and non-reactive pupils and hypotension, which may progress to circulatory failure.

INTRAVENOUS INDUCTION

In the UK an intravenous induction is performed for most cases. A potent short-acting hypnotic such as propofol, thiopental or etomidate is administered over 30 seconds. The required dose should be calculated based on the weight, but the requirement may vary and the effect of the dose being administered should be continuously assessed by observing the signs of loss of consciousness. With propofol, loss of consciousness is assessed by loss of verbal contact or dropping of a hand-held object. With thiopental the loss of the eyelash reflex is a reliable sign. A co-induction technique with a benzodiazepine or short-acting opioid is often chosen. The advantages include reduced anxiety, reduced requirements of the intravenous induction agent leading to reduced side-effects, and a reduced response to airway manoeuvres such as insertion of an airway.

With the loss of consciousness, typically breathing needs to be assisted because of brief apnoea. This can be done using a face-mask. Maintenance with inhalational agents is started at this stage. Usually a low concentration of inhalational agent is given with nitrous oxide (66%) and oxygen (33%); the concentration of the inhalational agent is rapidly increased using the 'overpressure' technique (see Chapter 2) to ensure that adequate levels are present in the central nervous system before the intravenous induction agent begins to be eliminated.

INHALATIONAL INDUCTION

The common indications for inhalational induction of anaesthesia are:

- children
- airway obstruction
- difficult venous access
- fear of needles.

Halothane or sevoflurane are suitable agents for inhalational induction. After preoxygenation, inhalation agents are added to the anaesthetic gases. In routine, elective cases the volatile agent is added to nitrous oxide and oxygen, but nitrous oxide is omitted if there is potential airway obstruction. Sevoflurane 8% can be added immediately, but halothane should be started at an inspired concentration of 0.5% and then increased by 0.5% every 3–4 breaths. The classic stages of anaesthesia including the excitatory phase should be anticipated. Adequate depth of anaesthesia (stage 3 – see above) must be ensured before airway procedures such as insertion of a laryngeal mask airway.

COMPLICATIONS

Common complications encountered with intravenous induction are:

- cardiovascular depression
- respiratory depression
- regurgitation or vomiting
- extravasation
- intra-arterial injection.

Cardiovascular depression is more common in the elderly, sick or in hypovolaemic patients. An intravenous infusion of fluids (for example 500 ml of crystalloid) usually helps. Ephedrine in small incremental doses (3 mg) may be required until the blood pressure is restored. The aim is to restore blood pressure to within ±20% of preoperative levels. Apnoea lasting for about 30 seconds is common, and breathing should be assisted during this period. Vomiting is an active process that cannot occur in the fully anaesthetized patient. Regurgitation is a passive process where the hydrostatic pressure of fluid and food in the stomach overcomes the resistance to flow up the oesophagus. It may be accompanied by aspiration through the laryngeal inlet and into the trachea.

Extravasation of the anaesthetic agent usually leads to swelling, pain or blanching around the site of injection. Tissue necrosis, especially if the solution is strongly alkaline such as thiopental, may occur. Hyaluronidase may be 'injected' down the same cannula to assist in dispersion of the extravasated drug. Intra-arterial injection is caused by injection of the induction agent into a cannula that has been placed in an artery by mistake. It is very painful (especially with thiopental). The injection should be stopped immediately and the cannula should be left in the artery and 5 ml of procaine 0.5% should be injected. Further treatment includes elevation of the limb, stellate ganglion block, brachial plexus block or sympathetic block. Accidental injection into an artery was common when these drugs were injected directly into a vein in the antecubital fossa; use of cannulae in veins on the hand or around the wrist has reduced this risk.

Airway complications of induction include:

- a prolonged excitatory phase
- airway obstruction
- laryngospasm
- bronchospasm
- hiccups.

Laryngeal spasm can occur if the airway is stimulated either by secretions of instrumentation during stage 2 or early stage 3. Further management of laryngospasm and bronchospasm is detailed in Action Plans 20 and 4 respectively. Hiccups usually subside with deepening anaesthesia.

Malignant hyperthermia

Volatile agents and succinylcholine are implicated in triggering malignant hyperthermia in susceptible individuals. See Action Plan 23.

MAINTENANCE OF ANAESTHESIA

After induction of anaesthesia and provision of an airway, the patient is prepared for surgery. Other lines such as arterial or central venous lines may be inserted, as may a nasogastric tube (experienced practitioners may insert this prior to intubation in a starved patient), a temperature probe, and a urinary catheter. If a combined general/regional or local anaesthetic technique is planned these may be done after induction (see Chapter 15).

Eye protection is of paramount importance. Usually the eyes are kept shut with tape. However, if the head is to be covered, or surgery is to be near the face or the patient has to be placed in the prone position, the eyes are given extra protection, for example with paraffin gauze, soft pads and wide tape to cover the whole eye and prevent surgical 'prep' solution entering the eyes. The patient is then positioned for surgery on the operating table and blankets or forced warm air devices are placed over the patient.

Movement to another position can lead to hypotension due to suppressed compensatory mechanisms under general anaesthesia. Changes in position should be performed slowly and with monitoring attached. Ensure plenty of help while positioning the patient. Patients must be securely held in whatever position they are placed in so that they cannot slip, and to prevent damage to the head and limbs which should be padded at pressure points or where nerves may be in danger of being compressed. Hyperextension or over-rotation of the neck and limbs should be avoided. Intermittent compression devices are placed around the calves for long procedures or where there are other increased risks of deep vein thrombosis.

MAINTENANCE TECHNIQUES

Irrespective of the technique of maintenance an adequate depth of anaesthesia should be ensured during surgery. The depth of anaesthesia is usually assessed by monitoring physiological signs in response to surgery.

The signs of light anaesthesia are:

- movement
- coughing
- tachypnoea
- increased sympathetic activity – tachycardia, hypertension, dilated pupils, sweating and tears.

Many of these 'warning' signs are absent in patients receiving a muscle relaxant. If anaesthesia is light, consider either increasing the amount of anaesthetic agent or increasing the amount of analgesia, or both. The signs of increased sympathetic activity can be masked by beta-blockers or other sympatholytic drugs. On the other hand, increased sympathetic stimulation can occur during hypoxia and hypercarbia. Surgical manoeuvres (such as anal stretch, cervical dilatation, stretching of the peritoneum) evoke intense autonomic activity which is usually short lasting. These manoeuvres require deeper planes of anaesthesia for a brief period of time. A short-acting opioid may be useful.

There are few absolute indications for either intravenous or inhalational maintenance. Intravenous anaesthesia may be more suitable when transferring patients in or outside the hospital. It is also useful when the airway is being shared, for example during rigid laryngoscopy. Either technique can be used in both spontaneously breathing patients or those receiving muscle relaxants and intermittent positive pressure ventilation (IPPV).

The choice of spontaneous ventilation versus the use of muscle relaxants and IPPV is made on the basis of a number of factors. Spontaneous ventilation usually through a laryngeal mask airway or other supraglottic device or via a face-mask is suitable for peripheral surgery, and where there is no other indication for muscle paralysis and the stomach is empty. The advantages of spontaneous ventilation are that depth of anaesthesia can be assessed more easily and there is less chance of awareness. The disadvantages are that respiration may be inadequate, or it may be compromised in certain positions. IPPV is usually achieved through a tracheal tube (or rarely a tracheostomy tube). IPPV can be performed through laryngeal mask airway providing the stomach is empty, the airway achieved is good and the inspiratory pressure is kept less than $20\,cmH_2O$. Surgery inside the abdominal or thoracic cavities, nearly all cases where tracheal intubation has been indicated (for example a shared airway during head and neck surgery), prolonged surgery or when control of the carbon dioxide partial pressure in the blood is important, require muscle paralysis and IPPV.

Intravenous anaesthesia

Maintenance of anaesthesia by continuous infusion of an intravenous agent is known as total intravenous anaesthesia (TIVA) and usually means infusion of propofol using the target controlled infusion technique (see Chapter 2). Propofol may be combined with nitrous oxide or infused with opioids such as remifentanil.

Maintenance of anaesthesia with volatile agents and spontaneous ventilation

The airway is usually maintained by a laryngeal mask airway or a face-mask and oral airway. Rarely a tracheal tube is considered for maintenance of airway. It is inserted using a short-acting muscle relaxant (succinylcholine) and manually ventilating the patient for 5–10 min until the succinylcholine wears off. The concentration of inhalational agent required to produce surgical anaesthesia depends on the type of surgery and the amount of analgesic and sedative drugs given. The dose of inhalational agent should be titrated to the patient's respiratory rate, heart rate, blood pressure and movement to surgery.

Maintenance of anaesthesia using muscle relaxants

With muscle relaxants, there will be no spontaneous movement of the patient or spontaneous respiratory pattern to indicate the depth of anaesthesia. Therefore, other indicators should be relied upon to ensure adequate depth and analgesia. The amount of analgesic drugs required depends on the extent of surgery and the patient's sympathetic response. If long-acting analgesics are used (for example morphine) then a pre-calculated dose should be given early on during surgery. This will prevent respiratory depression at the time of emergence. If TIVA is planned, then a combination of propofol and a short-acting analgesic (for example remifentanil) is given as a continuous infusion.

For controlled ventilation, the various parameters in adults are:

- Tidal volume: 9–12 ml/kg
- Respiratory rate: 10–15/minute
- Airway pressure: up to 25 cmH$_2$O
- I:E ratio: 1:1.5 or 1:2.

Increased airway pressure or difficulty in maintaining IPPV can occur with:

- airway obstruction
- kinking of the tube
- misplaced tube
- bronchial placement of tube
- bronchospasm
- surgical compression
- pneumothorax.

Decreased airway pressure usually indicates a disconnection. Ventilation can be assessed by inspecting chest movements, movement of the respiratory bag during spontaneous respiration, measuring the peak inspiratory pressure in mechanically ventilated patients, the capnograph, pulse oximeter, and, if needed, arterial blood gases.

Temperature control

Temperature is measured in all but the shortest cases (see Chapter 5). Most patients lose heat during anaesthesia. General anaesthesia inhibits the normal homeostatic mechanisms. Body cavities or exposed areas of body surface allow cooling in rooms that are usually maintained (except during surgery for neonates and infants) at a temperature comfortable for staff and not the patient. Covering up as much of the body as possible, in particular the head, warming intravenous fluids and using heat and moisture exchangers (HMEs) in breathing circuits will help. However, for most patients the only way to maintain normothermia is to use forced warm air blankets. Temperature measurement will also warn of overheating which can occur with this technique and will also help diagnose malignant hyperthermia (see Action Plan 23).

EMERGENCE FROM ANAESTHESIA

The aim is to change from the fully anaesthetized state to an awake, responsive, comfortable patient with intact airway reflexes and full muscle strength. The timing of stopping the hypnotic (inhalational or intravenous) agent is important. After stopping inhalational agents such as sevoflurane or desflurane, one can expect emergence within 3–5 minutes, while it may take about 5–10 minutes or more if one of the more soluble agents, such as isoflurane, is used.

> ⚠ **Many anaesthetists reduce the administration rate of the hypnotic prior to the end of surgery. Care must be taken to avoid awareness during this process.**

If used, muscle relaxants also take 2–3 minutes for complete reversal. Attempts at reversal must only begin when there is evidence of some spontaneous return of normal neuromuscular function – for example at least two twitches to a train-of-four stimulation. It is important not to reduce the hypnotic agent too early and before the return of full neuromuscular function as this may result in a paralysed patient who is otherwise awake, or a partially reversed patient who is struggling to maintain a patent airway and to breathe adequately. Once the patient is able to breathe adequately and the airway reflexes have returned, the tracheal tube should be removed. Extubation is a critical moment and, when performed in a lightly anaesthetized or partially awake patient, can lead to complications such as vomiting, coughing, and laryngospasm. An alternative to awake extubation is deep extubation. This is sometimes performed by experienced practitioners with the patient placed in the lateral position and still deeply anaesthetized. One indication is when coughing is to be avoided such as after middle ear surgery. Awake extubation is particularly indicated in the following conditions:

- full stomach
- difficult airway.

Following extubation oxygen is given by face-mask and if there is any airway obstruction an oral or nasal airway is inserted. However, an oral airway may lead to laryngeal stimulation and worsening of laryngospasm.

Laryngeal mask airways are removed when the patient has fully recovered – often in the recovery room. As a result of their relatively non-stimulating nature, patients often tolerate these airways until they are almost fully awake.

The causes of agitation during emergence include:

- hypoxia
- airway obstruction
- pain
- full bladder.

Delayed awakening is usually due to remaining anaesthetic agent or opioid. However, other causes are discussed in Action Plan 11.

RECOVERY FROM ANAESTHESIA

Any site where general or regional anaesthesia has been administered must be equipped with a suitable area to recover the patient. In most theatre complexes this is a recovery room. These are staffed by specially trained nurses or theatre practitioners, who care for patients on a 1:1 basis until their airway reflexes have fully recovered. Oxygen is administered to patients who have received general anaesthesia or sedation; observations including oxygen saturation, blood pressure and respiratory rate are recorded; pain relief is given if required; the surgical wound is inspected for bleeding etc; and the patient is prepared for return to the ward where there will be less intensive nursing care. An anaesthetist should always be readily available to care for patients who suffer a complication such as laryngospasm (see Chapter 16).

AIRWAY MANAGEMENT

Airway management is the most important aspect of anaesthetic practice. Mismanagement of the airway is a significant cause of adverse anaesthetic outcomes. Complete airway management includes a thorough evaluation and development of a management plan and an alternative plan in case the original fails.

ANATOMY

UPPER AIRWAY

The upper airway consists of the nasopharynx, the oropharynx, the hypopharynx and the larynx. The nasopharynx includes the nasal passages, septum, turbinates and adenoids. The oropharynx includes the oral cavity along with dentition, tongue, tonsils, and uvula.

LOWER AIRWAY

The lower airway starts at the vocal cords. In adults the vocal cords are the narrowest part of the airway. The larynx is composed of cartilages, ligaments and muscles. It is located at the level of the fourth to sixth cervical vertebrae. Its main functions include airway protection and phonation.

Amongst the cartilages of the larynx, there are three unpaired (single) cartilages and six paired cartilages. The unpaired cartilages are the thyroid, cricoid and epiglottis. The paired cartilages are the arytenoids, corniculates and cuneiforms. The thyroid cartilage is the largest cartilage and forms the main part of the anterior and lateral aspects of the body of the larynx. The cricoid cartilage is located inferior to the thyroid cartilage. It is the only complete cartilaginous ring in the airway. In children, the cricoid cartilage is the narrowest part of the airway. It is connected to the thyroid cartilage by the cricothyroid membrane which in adults is thin and has no blood vessels in the midline.

The laryngeal muscles perform three main functions:

- the posterior cricoarytenoid muscles open the glottis (abduction)
- the lateral cricoarytenoid muscles close the glottis (adduction)
- the cricothyroid, vocalis and thyroarytenoid muscles control the tension of vocal cords.

In adults the trachea is 12–15 cm long and is supported by C-shaped cartilages anteriorly, with a posterior membranous part which overlies the oesophagus. The first tracheal ring is anterior to the C6 vertebrae. The trachea ends at the level of the fifth thoracic vertebra where it bifurcates into the right and left main bronchi. The right main bronchus is larger than the left, and deviates from the vertical plane of the trachea at a less acute angle (25°) than the left main bronchus (45°). Aspirated material or an over-long tracheal tube is more likely to enter the right main bronchus than the left.

Innervation

The sensory innervation of the airway is provided by the glosso-pharyngeal nerve, the recurrent laryngeal nerve and the internal branch of the superior laryngeal nerve. The glossopharyngeal nerve supplies the posterior third of the tongue and the oropharynx. The internal branch of the superior laryngeal nerve (a branch of vagus nerve) supplies the mucosa from the epiglottis to the vocal cords. The recurrent laryngeal nerve (also a branch of the vagus nerve) supplies the mucosa below the vocal cords and the trachea. The motor supply to the larynx comes from the external branch of the superior laryngeal nerve and the recurrent laryngeal nerve.

AIRWAY EVALUATION

Details of airway evaluation are given in Chapter 6, Preoperative Assessment.

> ⚠️ It is important to remember that, at present, there is no single test that is either sensitive or specific in detecting a 'difficult airway'. Even a combination of the available tests fails to achieve this. Furthermore, an airway that is easy to maintain (with an oral airway and face-mask for example) may prove to be a difficult laryngoscopy and intubation, and the opposite – an airway difficult to maintain – may prove to be an easy intubation.

MANAGEMENT OF THE AIRWAY

PREOXYGENATION

The aim of preoxygenation is to replace the air in the functional residual capacity of the lungs with oxygen. This provides a reservoir of oxygen for uptake by blood after the onset of apnoea during anaesthetic induction. Under normal circumstances (breathing room air) desaturation (SaO_2 less than 90%) occurs after about

2 min of apnoea. However, after preoxygenation, (breathing oxygen for 3 min or four vital capacity breaths of oxygen over 30 seconds) the SaO_2 will remain more than 90% for 3–5 min. One end-point for preoxygenation is when the concentration of oxygen in the expired gas is >90%.

MAINTENANCE OF THE AIRWAY

The airway can be maintained using:

- a face-mask with or without an oral or nasal airway
- a laryngeal mask airway (or other supraglottic device)
- a tracheal tube or tracheostomy tube.

Table 10.1 lists equipment that should always be available whenever a general anaesthetic or other procedure that may result in loss of consciousness is undertaken.

TABLE 10.1 Equipment required for airway maintenance

Two laryngoscopes in working order with the blades of different sizes (standard and long)
Tracheal tubes – one of the calculated size and one a size smaller
Wire stillette
Gum elastic bougies or equivalent
Magill's forceps
Cuff inflation syringe
Securing tape or bandage
Catheter mount or angle-piece
Guedel airways in a range of sizes
Laryngeal mask airway in a range of sizes
Face-masks in a range of sizes
A suction source

(Emergency equipment – cricothyroidotomy kit, tracheostomy tubes, airway exchange catheters, fibreoptic laryngoscope and light source – should be available nearby, if needed)

FACE-MASK

The face-mask may be used:

- to preoxygenate a patient
- to assist or control ventilation after induction of anaesthesia prior to tracheal intubation
- for inhalational anaesthesia in spontaneously breathing patients for short operations.

Appropriate positioning of the patient's head and neck (see below) is important for successful face-mask airway maintenance. A face-mask is selected to provide a snug fit around the bridge of the nose, cheeks and mouth. Disposable clear plastic masks have the advantage over traditional black rubber masks that they allow observation of the lips and mouth (detection of cyanosis, regurgitation or vomiting) during airway management and a guarantee of cleanliness. The mask is placed on the patient's face and is held in place with one or two hands (Figure 10.1). The little finger is used to support the angle of the mandible, the third and fourth fingers support the body of the mandible, and the index finger and thumb are used to apply firm pressure on the mask. Experienced practitioners can often manage the airway with one hand and control (squeeze) the reservoir bag with the other. If both hands are used to hold the mask an assistant is asked to control the reservoir bag. Holding the mask with two hands allows an effective jaw thrust to be applied in case of upper airway obstruction. In some patients who are either edentulous or are large or have a beard, achieving a tight seal around the mask with one hand can be difficult.

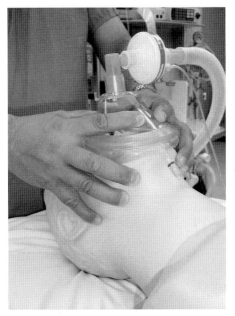

Fig. 10.1 Two handed technique to hold face-mask and perform a jaw thrust.

After the induction of anaesthesia, the muscles of the upper airway lose their tone, causing the tongue to fall back onto the soft palate and posterior pharyngeal wall, leading to airway obstruction. Airway obstruction during spontaneous ventilation may be recognized by:

- stridor
- paradoxical movement of chest and abdomen (during inspiration the abdomen protrudes out while the chest is drawn in)
- very small or no respiratory excursions in the reservoir bag if breathing spontaneously.

Airway patency can be restored by:

- a chin lift producing neck extension
- a jaw thrust
- insertion of a Guedel's oral airway
- insertion of a nasal airway.

The correct size of airway must be used (see Equipment, Chapter 4). An oral airway should only be inserted after the patient has been adequately anaesthetized (stage 3, see Chapter 9) as insertion in a lightly anaesthetized patient can cause vomiting, laryngospasm and dental trauma. Oral airways should be inserted the wrong way up until the tip of the airway is over the back of the tongue when it should be rotated 180° to the correct orientation (Figure 10.2).

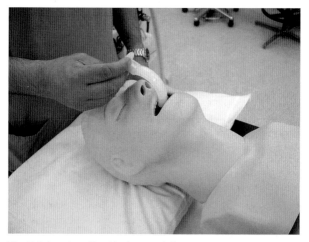

Fig. 10.2 Insertion of 'upside down' oral airway.

A nasal airway is better tolerated by awake or sedated patients with an intact gag reflex. However, they can cause epistaxis and may not be as effective as an oral airway. They should be avoided in patients with fractures of the base of the skull.

In patients who are apnoeic or who have received a muscle relaxant, a face-mask with or without an airway is used to provide intermittent positive pressure lung inflation. In healthy subjects, airway pressures should not exceed 25 cmH$_2$O during positive pressure lung inflation. However, if greater pressures are required or if the lung inflation is inadequate, other methods of maintaining the airway should be considered, such as a laryngeal mask airway or tracheal tube. The complications of using a face-mask include pressure injuries to the soft tissue around the mouth, nose, lips and eyes. Face-mask airway maintenance does not protect the lower airway from the aspiration of gastric contents.

LARYNGEAL MASK AIRWAY

The laryngeal mask airway comes in various sizes (see Equipment, Chapter 4). Insertion may cause a reflex reaction to stimulation of the structures of the oropharynx and laryngopharynx and intravenous induction with propofol is usually recommended as it rapidly inhibits the laryngeal reflexes. Once the patient is adequately anaesthetized (after loss of consciousness and the cessation of voluntary movements) the laryngeal mask airway can be inserted over the tongue and advanced until it is seated behind the larynx (see Figure 10.3). The cuff is then inflated. Non-obstructed spontaneous ventilation by the patient or successful positive pressure ventilation of the lungs in apnoeic patients indicates proper positioning.

The laryngeal mask airway can be used to establish an airway when the tracheal intubation is difficult due to poor visualization of the larynx, and it may also be used as a guide for placement of a tracheal tube. The laryngeal mask airway does not protect the airway against regurgitation or pulmonary aspiration. Therefore, it should be used only in patients who are not at risk of regurgitation. The laryngeal mask airway has been used to provide intermittent positive pressure ventilation of the lungs in suitable patients.

Complications of laryngeal mask airway use:

- airway obstruction – this is usually due to malpositioning of the laryngeal mask airway or it pushing the epiglottis forwards against the laryngeal inlet
- laryngospasm

- coughing
- bronchospasm
- gastro-oesophageal reflux
- sore throat
- transient changes in vocal cord function.

  Contraindications to laryngeal mask airway use:

- limited mouth opening
- patients suspected of having a full stomach
- hiatus hernia
- gastro-oesophageal reflux
- intestinal obstruction
- morbid obesity
- poor lung compliance
- increased airway resistance.

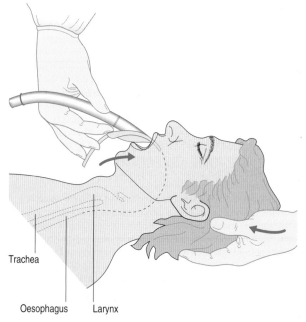

Trachea

Oesophagus   Larynx

Fig. 10.3 a. Technique for insertion of laryngeal mask airway. Courtesy of Intavent Orthofix Ltd.

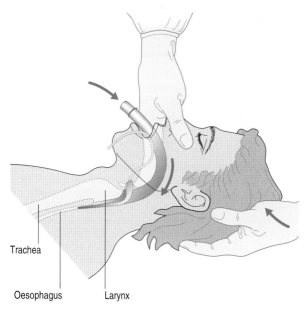

Trachea

Oesophagus   Larynx

Fig. 10.3 b. Technique for insertion of laryngeal mask airway (Cont'd).
Courtesy of Intavent Orthofix Ltd.

TRACHEAL INTUBATION

Tracheal intubation provides the most reliable patent airway, especially when patients are at risk of aspiration. Other indications include:

- difficult airway maintenance by face-mask or laryngeal mask airway
- prolonged anaesthesia
- controlled ventilation
- surgery around head and neck
- surgery inside the thorax or abdomen
- any other requirement for a paralysed, ventilated patient.

Typically, tracheal intubation is performed with a laryngoscope. The curved Macintosh laryngoscope is most commonly used (see Equipment, Chapter 4). The blades range in size from No. 1 to No. 4, with most adult patients requiring a No. 3 blade.

Technique of laryngoscopy and tracheal intubation

The patient is positioned supine with the head resting on a pillow, in the so-called 'sniffing the morning air position' (flexion of the lower cervical spine and extension of the head at atlanto-occipital junction [upper cervical spine]) (Figure 10.4). This position aligns the oral, pharyngeal and laryngeal axis so that the pathway from the lips to the glottis is nearly a straight line. The laryngoscope is held in the left hand, whilst the right hand is used to stabilize the head and open the mouth. The laryngoscope is inserted into the right side of the patient's mouth avoiding the incisor teeth and pushing the tongue to the left. The tip of the blade is advanced in the midline over the back of the tongue until the epiglottis comes into view. The tip of a Macintosh laryngoscope blade should be positioned above the epiglottis, into the vallecula (the space between the base of the tongue and the epiglottis). The tongue and pharyngeal soft tissues are then lifted, pulling the epiglottis up without directly touching it, exposing the glottic opening. You should use your arm and shoulder to lift the laryngoscope handle in an anterior and forward direction (along the long axis of the handle containing the batteries). The tendency to lever the laryngoscope against the upper incisor teeth or upper gum should be avoided to prevent trauma.

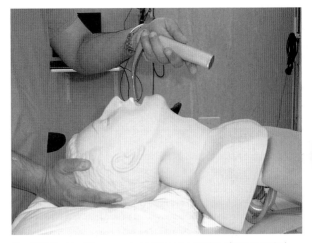

Fig. 10.4 Flexion of lower cervical spine and extension of upper cervical spine to produce optimal position for tracheal intubation.

The Miller blade, which is straight, is less commonly used. The tip of the Miller blade is passed beneath the laryngeal surface of the epiglottis and the epiglottis itself is then lifted to expose the vocal cords. There is more risk of trauma to the epiglottis and stimulation of the laryngeal surface of the epiglottis.

The size of the tracheal tube used depends on the patient's age and body build. Usually an 8.0 mm internal diameter cuffed tube is used for women and a 9.0 mm tube for men. The tube is held in the right hand as one would hold a pencil and advanced through the oral cavity through the right corner of the mouth and then through the vocal cords. External pressure on the cricoid or thyroid cartilage may be required to help visualize the laryngeal inlet. The proximal end of the tube cuff is placed so that the cuff is below the vocal cords, and the length markings on the tube are noted in relation to patient's lips. The cuff is inflated to obtain a seal in the presence of 20–30 cmH$_2$O pressure of gas in the breathing system.

The next step is to verify the position of the tracheal tube. The best method to determine the position of the tube is by detection of carbon dioxide in expired gas. It is possible for gas in the stomach to contain carbon dioxide but this will only be present in the first few 'breaths'. Visualization of the end of the tube advancing through the vocal cords is also taken as a sign of correct placement. However, tubes may be displaced after 'correct' insertion. Auscultation of both lung fields in the axilla and over the stomach may also be used to confirm correct placement, but is less reliable. Asymmetrical breath sounds may indicate that the tip of the tube lies in one or other of the main bronchi (usually the right – see above). The tube should be withdrawn until breath sounds are heard bilaterally.

Complications of orotracheal intubation include:

- injury to the lips, tongue or teeth
- injury to larynx (especially the arytenoid cartilages and the vocal cords)
- tracheal mucosa tear
- sympathetic stimulation.

Attempting laryngoscopy or tracheal intubation in lightly anaesthetized patients who are not fully relaxed can result in laryngospasm, coughing, and bronchospasm. The laryngoscope should be removed, face-mask ventilation should be continued and anaesthesia deepened or more muscle relaxant given to achieve adequate conditions. A peripheral nerve stimulator can be used to ensure complete neuromuscular blockade before commencing laryngoscopy and intubation.

Nasotracheal intubation

Nasotracheal intubation is indicated in patients undergoing procedures inside the mouth. Compared with orally placed tracheal tubes, the maximum diameter is usually smaller and the tubes longer, leading to increased resistance.

The contraindications to the use of a nasal tube include:

- fracture of the base of the skull
- nasal fractures
- nasal polyps
- coagulopathy.

A vasoconstrictor such as phenylephrine–lidocaine mixture may be applied to the nasal mucosa. Usually a size 7.0 mm tube is used for women and a size 8.0 mm for men. The right nostril is preferred because the bevel of most tracheal tubes when introduced through the right nostril faces the flat nasal septum, reducing the chance of damage to the turbinates. After passage through the nose into the pharynx, the tube is advanced through the laryngeal inlet under direct vision using a laryngoscope and Magill's forceps to direct the tip of the tube towards the laryngeal opening. The complications are similar to those described for oral tracheal intubation. In addition, nasal haemorrhage, submucosal tear and dislodgement of tonsils or adenoids may also occur. Infection of the frontal and maxillary sinuses and bacteraemia can occur after long-term nasotracheal intubation.

AWAKE INTUBATION

The indications for awake (oral or nasal) intubation include an anticipated difficult intubation in a patient at risk of aspiration and uncertainty about the ability to ventilate the lungs or intubate the trachea following induction of general anaesthesia (due to anatomical abnormalities, cervical spine disease, restricted mouth opening, skin contractures around the neck, obesity, laryngeal or mediastinal tumours, retrosternal goitre).

To perform an awake intubation the upper airway must be anaesthetized topically. Lidocaine may be applied by spray or topically to the nose or anterior oropharnx, a 4% lidocaine gargle or nebulizer is used to anaesthetize the rest of the airway above the larynx. Bilateral superior laryngeal nerve blocks may also be used to anaesthetize supraglottic structures. Further lidocaine is 'injected' down the suction channel of the fibreoptic laryngoscope once the tip has passed the vocal cords. Alternatively, a transtracheal injection of local anaesthetic can be used to anaesthetize the glottis and upper trachea. A 20 gauge needle is inserted through the cricothyroid membrane in the midline. After aspiration of air to confirm placement within the tracheal lumen, 2 ml of 2% lidocaine is injected and the needle is withdrawn quickly; such injection of lidocaine can cause severe coughing.

FIBREOPTIC INTUBATION

The flexible fibreoptic laryngoscope can be used when direct laryngoscopy is unable to provide an adequate view. This can be used to intubate patients when they are anaesthetized or awake (after adequate topical anaesthesia). The standard equipment for fibreoptic intubation includes an oral bite block, topical anaesthetics, suction equipment and a sterile flexible fibreoptic laryngoscope with a light source. A lubricated tracheal tube is placed (preloaded) over the fibreoptic laryngoscope. The laryngoscope is advanced towards the laryngeal inlet through either the nose or mouth. Once the tip of the layrngoscope is in the trachea, the tracheal tube is slid off the laryngoscope and into the trachea.

The usual checks for correct placement are made. Identification of the carina beyond the aperture of the tracheal tube assists in confirming correct placement.

Successful awake fibreoptic laryngoscopy requires adequate patient preparation, a cooperative patient and knowledge of airway anatomy to recognize the main structures as they are encountered. The technique is usually taught to trainees in the later stages of their training.

PERCUTANEOUS CRICOTHYROTOMY

This is an emergency airway technique, in a 'cannot intubate, cannot ventilate' situation. A large bore (14 gauge) cannula is placed through the cricothyroid membrane into the trachea. Oxygen is then administered by connecting the cannula to a source of high pressure oxygen with an on/off control. Once in place, the catheter must be carefully held in position. Dislodgement during ventilation may lead to severe barotrauma, emphysema of the neck and anterior chest and loss of the airway. Although oxygen can be forced into the trachea and lungs with this technique a route for exhalation is not provided. If there is complete or near complete upper airway obstruction severe barotrauma of the lungs may occur. Oxygenation, but not ventilation, can be achieved with this technique and it is only a temporary manoeuvre allowing life-saving oxygenation. Larger diameter cannulae have become available that may allow connection to a routine anaesthetic circuit and permit some exhalation. They are either inserted as cannulae (with a sharp introducer/stylet) or using a guide-wire inserted through a narrow needle used to 'guide' the wider airway through the cricothyroid membrane.

RAPID SEQUENCE INDUCTION

This is indicated in patients at risk of aspiration and includes those who have recently eaten, pregnant patients, and those with bowel obstruction, morbid obesity or symptomatic reflux. Rapid sequence intubation requires the administration of neuromuscular blocking drugs without first verifying that face-mask ventilation is possible, introducing another risk (although reducing the risk of aspiration). As this risk is combined with the other risks of succinylcholine use, such as anaphylaxis, muscle pains and hyperkalaemia, this technique should only be used when necessary. If there is any doubt that intubation may be difficult, an alternative technique such as awake intubation should be considered.

Equipment necessary for rapid sequence induction:

- suction
- several different laryngoscopes and different sizes of blades
- tracheal tubes of various sizes
- a trained assistant who can apply effective cricoid pressure
- bougies and laryngeal masks
- a tipping trolley or bed.

The lungs are preoxygenated (see above). The head and neck are placed into the standard intubation position and the assistant identifies the cricoid cartilage. A pre-calculated dose of an induction agent (usually thiopental, propofol or etomidate) is administered over 10–30 seconds. This is followed immediately by succinylcholine (1.5 mg/kg). Simultaneously, the assistant places firm downward pressure on the cricoid cartilage to compress and occlude the oesophagus. This manoeuvre reduces the risk of passive regurgitation of gastric contents into the pharynx and may bring the vocal cords into a better view by displacing them posteriorly. It will not prevent active vomiting. No attempt is made to ventilate the lungs by mask, but intubation is performed after 60 seconds, when all muscle fasciculation due to the succinylcholine has stopped. Cricoid pressure is maintained until successful tracheal intubation is verified and the tube cuff has been inflated. If intubation attempts are unsuccessful, cricoid pressure is maintained continuously during all subsequent intubation manoeuvres and while face-mask ventilation is in progress. The patient is placed in a head-down position. A decision must be made rapidly as to whether the procedure *must* continue. In nearly all situations the patient can be allowed to awaken whilst help is summoned and other options are explored. If face-mask ventilation is impossible, placement of laryngeal mask airway may provide an adequate airway. If an airway still can not be established, cricoid pressure may be released or a cricothyroidotomy performed (see Action Plan 10).

FLUID AND ELECTROLYTE BALANCE

Approximately 60% of the total body weight is water. Thus, in an adult weighing 70 kg, there are approximately 42 litres of water. Of this water, two-thirds (28 L) is in the intracellular compartment, and one-third (14 L) is distributed in the extracellular compartments. In a healthy adult, the total blood volume is ~5 L of which 2 L are occupied by red cells and the rest is plasma. In adults the total blood volume can be estimated as 75 ml per kg of body weight.

Amongst the ions, sodium is distributed mainly extracellularly, whilst potassium is mainly intracellular. Albumin is the most important oncotic molecule in the extracellular fluid. Its concentration in blood is ~40 g/litre. The extracellular fluid and its composition is regulated by aldosterone, anti-diuretic hormone and atrial natriuretic peptide.

SODIUM BALANCE

Sodium maintains the osmolality of plasma and is an important ion in creation of the action potential in excitable tissues. Hyponatraemia is usually due to an increase in total body water rather than a decrease in total body sodium. Treatment of hyponatraemia is fluid restriction and use of isotonic solutions such as normal saline for maintenance. Hypertonic saline solutions are rarely required. The aim is to correct the serum sodium slowly. Hypernatraemia is often the result of excessive infusion of sodium in chronic fluid therapies. Other causes include:

- diabetes insipidus
- excess use of osmotic diuretics
- failure of water intake (as in coma)
- increased water loss due to fever or hyperventilation
- vomiting.

If hypernatraemia is due to water loss, then 5% glucose should be used. Diabetes insipidus should be controlled with vasopressin supplements.

POTASSIUM BALANCE

Potassium is an important intracellular ion, and maintains the transmembrane potential.

The causes of hypokalaemia include:

- Redistribution into intracellular compartment – e.g. insulin administration, alkalosis.

- Loss of potassium – diarrhoea, vomiting, nasogastric secretions and fistulae.
- Excess renal excretion – diuretic therapy, hyperaldosteronism, and renal failure (diuretic phase).

Acute hypokalaemia causes muscle weakness and ventricular dysrhythmias; chronic hypokalaemia is much better tolerated. As a guide, a plasma deficit of 1 mmol/l equates to a total potassium loss of about 100–200 mmol. Precipitating factors should be corrected and potassium chloride solutions administered slowly. The maximum recommended rate is 10 mmol/h; however, in severe hypokalaemia infusions of up to 20 mmol/h can be given with ECG monitoring.

The commonest causes of hyperkalaemia are renal failure, metabolic acidosis, massive blood transfusion and extensive tissue damage. The early ECG findings are tall T-waves and a shortened QT interval. When the plasma concentration of potassium exceeds 8 mmol/l, the QRS complex becomes widened, and ventricular fibrillation may occur spontaneously. See Chapter 17 for emergency treatment of hyperkalaemia.

ASSESSMENT OF FLUID STATUS

Mild dehydration can be diagnosed by assessing skin texture and general well-being. Hypovolaemia can be present despite a normal blood pressure. Up to 10% of total body water can be lost without significant clinical features. More than 10% of fluid loss leads to postural hypotension. Tachycardia, hypotension and oliguria indicate significant fluid loss. Metabolic acidosis, raised haematocrit and urea indicate significant dehydration. During anaesthesia the signs of fluid loss may be masked by other events or co-morbidity. Patients who are particularly at risk of major fluid shifts, undergoing major thoracic or abdominal surgery or after major trauma for example, should have a central venous pressure line inserted prior to the commencement of surgery.

MAINTENANCE REQUIREMENTS

For an adult, the maintenance requirement of water is approximately 1–2 ml/kg/h. To calculate the initial maintenance requirement, one should include the fasting time. Therefore, a patient of 70 kg body weight who has fasted for 6 hours before the anaesthetic will require about 500–700 ml of crystalloid solution over the first hour followed by 100 ml/h thereafter. The requirement for sodium is approximately 75–100 mmol/day and the requirement for potassium is 40–80 mmol/day. Other ions such as magnesium, calcium and phosphate do not require replacement in the short-term. However, patients on long-term intravenous fluid therapy may require replacement of these ions. In children the formula 4 ml/kg/h for the first 10 kg of body weight, plus 2 ml/kg/h for the next 10 kg of body weight, plus 1 ml/kg/h body weight thereafter is appropriate.

REPLACEMENT REQUIREMENTS

In addition to maintenance fluid, extra fluid may be required to replace:

- surgical losses – blood, evaporation from open wounds or cavities (up to 1 l/h from the abdomen)
- evaporative loss from skin (especially burns)
- GI loss (fistula, vomiting and diarrhoea)
- 'third space' loss (severe tissue injury or surgical oedema).

Fluids should also be replaced to match physiological losses in the urine, gastric secretions and intestinal secretions. Normal saline is normally used for replacement fluid.

Evaporative loss

Evaporative loss depends on the type of surgery and the body area it exposes to the atmosphere. Body cavity surgeries, such as abdominal surgery and thoracic surgery, are associated with an increased amount of evaporative loss. Typically, for minor surgeries, 2 ml/kg/hour should be given, and for major surgery, including body cavities, 4–6 ml/kg/hour of crystalloid solution should be given.

Third space loss

Fluid is 'lost' in tissue oedema which may be extensive in patients with trauma or undergoing major surgery. Up to 6 ml/kg/hour may be required.

BLOOD LOSS

Blood loss should be assessed by checking the suction bottle (allow for fluid used for flushing or irrigation), weighing swabs and by inspecting the floor and drapes for blood loss. Also, haematocrit can be measured to assess blood loss. Clinically, heart rate, blood pressure, urine output and central venous pressure can be measured to get an idea of blood loss. A patient with no pre-existing medical illness, and normal haemoglobin levels can lose up to 10% of total blood volume (for a healthy adult this equates to ~500 ml). Signs of blood loss such as hypotension, tachycardia, reduced urine output and acidosis start after 15% of total blood volume has been lost. Blood loss of less than 20% of estimated total blood volume is usually treated with crystalloid or colloid (see below) infusions. The exact trigger for starting blood transfusion depends on a number of factors including the preoperative haemoglobin, the expected rate of continuing blood loss, the presence of co-morbidity such as ischaemic heart disease, and the use of intraoperative and postoperative cell-salvage techniques. Fit healthy patients without ongoing losses should only be transfused if it is predicted the haemoglobin will be less than 9 g/dl. Once blood replacement is more than half the blood volume, the coagulation profile should be investigated for dilutional coagulopathy and thrombocytopaenia.

INTRAVENOUS FLUIDS

COLLOIDS

Colloids are solutions of large molecules which have an oncotic pressure – the molecules do not normally cross the endothelial barrier and enter the tissues or intracellular spaces.

Colloids (Gelofusine®, Haemaccel®, human albumin solution, and hydroxyethyl starch solutions) are used to expand the plasma volume. In conditions that cause leaky capillaries (burns and sepsis) these fluids, along with their large molecules, may spread throughout the body. The proteins in Gelofusine® and Haemaccel® are rapidly metabolized, after which these solutions act as crystalloids.

The advantages of using colloids are:

- reduced tissue oedema
- reduced cerebral oedema
- plasma expander.

The disadvantages are:

- allergic reactions
- pulmonary oedema in cases of capillary leak
- coagulopathy if more than 1–2 L is infused.

CRYSTALLOIDS

The electrolyte composition of different crystalloid solutions is given in Table 11.1. Glucose (dextrose) is rapidly metabolized and solutions containing glucose soon act as if they are hypotonic. Glucose solutions should only be used when there is a risk of overloading the body with sodium. Although the requirements for sodium are modest, most patients can handle greater quantities, and are at risk of hyponatraemia if large volumes of glucose containing solutions are given. If crystalloids are used to replace lost blood, it is necessary to infuse 2–3 times the volume lost as the majority of the fluid given is rapidly transferred to the extravascular compartment as the endothelial barrier is fully permeable to ions in these solutions.

The disadvantages of crystalloid infusions are:

- after blood loss, the haemodynamic improvement is short-lived
- peripheral oedema.

TABLE 11.1 Composition of crystalloid solutions	
Solution	Electrolyte composition (mmol/l)
Hartmann's solution (compound sodium lactate)	Sodium 131 Chloride 112 Potassium 5 Calcium 4 HCO_3 29 (as lactate)
Normal saline (0.9% NaCl)	Sodium 154 Chloride 154
5% glucose	No electrolytes
Dextrose saline (4% Glucose and 0.18% NaCl)	Sodium 31 Chloride 31

ANAESTHESIA FOR THE SURGICAL SPECIALITIES

Details on anaesthesia for obstetrics, cardiac surgery, neurosurgery and spinal surgery are beyond the scope of this book.

ABDOMINAL SURGERY

Abdominal surgery ranges from minor surgery for hernia repair or external perineal surgery to major large intestine resections and surgery to the upper gastrointestinal tract and liver. Anaesthetic considerations for emergency surgery are dealt with elsewhere.

PHYSIOLOGICAL CONSIDERATIONS

Oesophagus

The lower oesophageal sphincter is the major barrier to gastro-oesophageal reflux. A number of conditions are associated with decreased lower oesophageal sphincter tone:

- obesity
- hiatus hernia
- pregnancy
- oesophageal disease.

The lower oesophageal sphincter tone is also reduced by some drugs:

- anticholinergics – atropine, glycopyrrolate
- opioids
- inhaled anaesthetics
- intravenous induction agents.

Stomach

The stomach produces approximately 2 L of secretions in a day and the pH is between 1 and 3.5. The ingestion of clear fluids up to 2 h before induction of anaesthesia does not increase the volume of gastric fluid in otherwise healthy patients undergoing elective surgery procedures. Factors that influence the rate of gastric emptying are given in Table 12.1.

Small intestine

The mucosa of the small intestine secretes 5–6 L of fluid in a day; about 80–90% of this fluid is reabsorbed. The motility of the small intestine is increased by stimulation of the parasympathetic nervous system or by parasympathomimetic drugs, and is decreased

TABLE 12.1 Factors that affect gastric emptying

Cause	Increased gastric emptying	Decreased gastric emptying
Physiological	Gastric distension	Pregnancy Acid High protein food
Diseases	Thyrotoxicosis	Anxiety Shock Pain Diabetes mellitus Sepsis Intestinal obstruction
Drugs	Neostigmine Nicotine Metoclopramide	Alcohol Anticholinergics Opioids Anaesthetics

by intestinal distension, bowel manipulation, and stimulation of the sympathetic nervous system.

ANAESTHESIA

Tracheal intubation protects the upper airway against aspiration of gastric contents in patients at risk of reflux. Regional anaesthesia may be used alone for abdominal wall surgery such as inguinal hernia repair or perineal surgery, but for upper abdominal surgery a high block (T4) is needed and is not well tolerated. For most abdominal procedures general anaesthesia is used and may be combined with a regional technique. This approach has the advantage of providing good surgical conditions with adequate muscle relaxation and the analgesia can be extended in the postoperative period. The good pain relief provided by an epidural block helps to restore ventilatory function in the postoperative period, especially after abdominal surgery, and therefore reduces postoperative chest complications.

Conduct of general anaesthesia

Rapid sequence induction is indicated in patients with a 'full stomach'. Muscle relaxation is required for most intra-abdominal surgery. The use of nitrous oxide is relatively contraindicated in bowel obstruction, or during anastomosis of an unprepared bowel. This is because nitrous oxide is more soluble than nitrogen and diffuses into the bowel lumen faster than nitrogen can diffuse out.

Intraluminal gas volume can double within about 10 min of 60% nitrous oxide inhalation. The resulting distension can interfere with surgery and may also impair the perfusion of the obstructed bowel.

Administration of fluids for maintenance and replacement of deficits and ongoing losses is essential (see Chapter 11). Evaporative losses from the peritoneal surfaces can be as much as 8 ml/kg/h.

Nasogastric tube

Nasogastric tubes are usually inserted prior to anaesthesia in patients with trauma or bowel obstruction. Suction via large bore nasogastric tube can reduce the volume of gastric air and contents. They do not, however, guarantee an empty stomach. The presence of a nasogastric tube can compromise the seal around a facemask and, in theory, compromises the efficiency of the lower oesophageal sphincter. However, cricoid pressure *is* effective in the presence of a nasogastric tube. For elective upper abdominal surgery nasogastric tubes are placed after induction of anaesthesia. Complications of nasogastric tube insertion include bleeding, nasal submucosal disruption and incorrect placement (into the trachea).

Insertion of a nasogastric tube is contraindicated in patients with a suspected fracture of the base of the skull or trauma to the nose; an orogastric tube should be used instead.

INTRAOPERATIVE PROBLEMS

Circulatory effects of bowel manipulation

Hypotension, tachycardia and skin flushing can occur during bowel manipulation. This may herald the onset of sepsis. However, in most cases these changes are transient and require the infusion of fluids and, occasionally, vasopressors.

Temperature control

Heat loss is common during abdominal surgery. The exposed peritoneal surface causes evaporative as well as convective heat loss. The temperature should be monitored, and active measures should be taken to maintain the core temperature >36°C. These measures include use of warmed intravenous fluids and warm air blankets.

Deterioration of lung function

The use of retractors, packs around the liver and diaphragm, the head-down position (Trendelenberg) and insufflation of carbon dioxide gas during laparoscopic surgery can compromise lung

function. The elevation of the diaphragm and decrease in functional residual capacity cause hypoventilation and hypoxaemia,
particularly in spontaneously breathing patients. Intermittent
positive pressure ventilation and positive end expiratory pressure
(PEEP) should be used in these circumstances.

Hiccups

Hiccups occur spontaneously or in response to stimulation of the
diaphragm or abdominal viscera. The following measures may be
used to control hiccups:

- increase the depth of anaesthesia
- passage of a nasogastric tube
- aspiration of gas from the stomach
- increase the degree of neuromuscular blockade.

Faecal contamination

Contamination from a perforation of the gut can cause peritonitis
and sepsis. The patient should be managed with the placement
of central venous pressure and arterial pressure monitoring,
aggressive fluid therapy and the use of inotropes if necessary.
Admission to the HDU or ICU is usually required. At the end of
the procedure the trachea should be extubated only if the patient is
haemodynamically stable and gas exchange is adequate.

ANAESTHETIC CONSIDERATIONS FOR SPECIFIC SURGERIES

Perineal surgery

Drainage of ischiorectal abscess, haemorrhoidectomy, and surgery
for anal fissure are relatively brief procedures. Patients are usually
in the lithotomy position. Deep planes of general anaesthesia
are necessary transiently during stretching of the anal sphincter.
Tracheal intubation is required for patients undergoing general
anaesthesia in the prone position. Caudal epidural block can be
helpful for postoperative analgesia after anal surgery.

Hernia repair

For inguinal or femoral hernia repairs, either regional or general anaesthesia can be used. Ilioinguinal (field) block is often
performed for analgesia. Retraction of the peritoneum or of the
spermatic cord can be unpleasant and produce a profound vagal
response during regional anaesthesia. For elective surgery general
anaesthesia with a laryngeal mask airway is usually satisfactory.

Large intestine resections

These are major operations requiring careful fluid balance maintenance, temperature control, and provision of good postoperative analgesia (often by epidural analgesia). Patients may have received bowel 'prep' making them dehydrated or have an acute abdomen with fluid loss due to vomiting or diarrhoea. Adequate preoperative fluid resuscitation is essential.

Laparoscopic surgery

See section on laparoscopic procedures in gynaecological surgery section.

POSTOPERATIVE CARE

Patients who have undergone major abdominal surgery should be admitted to an area capable of managing epidural infusions and complicated fluid balance. This is often the High Dependency Unit.

DENTAL AND MAXILLO-FACIAL SURGERY

Many of the considerations about a shared airway and intra- and postoperative bleeding into the airway are the same as for ENT surgery (below).

ENT SURGERY

Anaesthesia for ENT surgery often requires sharing the airway with the surgeon, or at least having the surgeon operating on the head, which will be 'out-of-bounds' for the anaesthetist. In addition patients may have a difficult airway and a thorough airway assessment is essential to detect potential airway obstruction or difficult intubation.

EAR SURGERY

Ear surgery ranges from the very straightforward such as grommet insertion to prolonged procedures such as cochlear implants. Except for grommet insertion, nitrous oxide is avoided in middle ear surgery as a change in pressure in the middle ear cavity can be harmful to the tympanic membrane or grafts. PONV is common after middle ear surgery.

SURGERY ON THE NOSE AND ORAL CAVITY

Bleeding from the nasal mucosa may be profuse and can contaminate the airway during and after the operation. A vasoconstrictor, such as cocaine paste, is usually applied to the nasal mucosa by the surgeon before the start of surgery. Because of the vascularity of the nasal mucosa, these drugs can be rapidly absorbed and give rise to systemic changes.

 A throat pack is usually used intraoperatively and must be removed prior to extubation.

Other problems with intra-oral or nasal surgery include:

- kinking of the tracheal tube with airway instrumentation
- swallowed blood
- blood loss in children.

Tonsillectomy is not as common as it was. In adults it can be painful postoperatively.

DIRECT LARYNGOSCOPY AND LARYNGEAL SURGERY

Direct laryngoscopy is performed for diagnostic purposes or for microlaryngeal surgery. Many patients will often have undergone awake nasendoscopy by the surgeon prior to surgery and reference to these findings should help plan the anaesthetic.

If the history, examination or investigations suggest airway obstruction, an inhalational induction should be contemplated. You must call for senior help.

Major laryngeal surgery is usually performed for malignant lesions and involves extensive dissection of the neck. It is beyond the scope of this book.

GYNAECOLOGICAL SURGERY

The general principles of anaesthesia for gynaecological procedures are similar to those for abdominal surgery. The incidence of PONV is high after pelvic surgery and the use of prophylactic anti-emetics is routine. Deep vein thrombosis is also common and patients likely to be immobilized require prophylactic measures including compression devices, stockings and low-molecular weight heparin.

DILATATION AND CURETTAGE (D&C); EVACUATION OF RETAINED PRODUCTS OF CONCEPTION (ERPC), SUCTION TERMINATION OF PREGNANCY (TOP)

Preoperative considerations

- Some members of staff may not agree to participate on religious grounds; these values should be respected and alternative staff arranged.
- Assume a full stomach in emergency cases, or in patients beyond the first trimester of pregnancy.

Intraoperative considerations

- Rapid sequence induction if there is risk of full stomach.
- Volatile agents may cause uterine relaxation and bleeding; restrict their use to concentrations of less than or equal to 1.3 MAC.
- Intravenous ergometrine may cause hypertension; oxytocin may cause hypotension.

HYSTEROSCOPY

Hysteroscopy is usually performed with general anaesthesia. Alternatively, the surgeon can administer a paracervical or intra-cervical block. Instrumentation of the uterus may lead to uterine perforation and haemorrhage.

The use of fluids for uterine distension can cause fluid over-load, hyponatraemia and DIC (similar to TURP surgery). Use of carbon dioxide for uterine distension may be associated with a gas leak from the fallopian tubes leading to abdominal distension and hypercarbia. There is also a risk of gas embolism.

LAPAROSCOPIC PROCEDURES

General anaesthesia with tracheal intubation and mechanical ventilation is the most accepted technique. However, in selected patients, mechanical ventilation or spontaneous breathing via a laryngeal mask airway may be used. Most procedures are done as day cases. Local anaesthesia can be instilled around the fallopian tubes after laparoscopic sterilization. Shoulder tip pain indicates residual abdominal gas irritating the diaphragm.

The following problems may be associated with laparoscopic procedures:

- Hypoventilation due to increased intra-abdominal pressure, hypercarbia and absorption of carbon dioxide.
- Hypertension during peritoneal insufflation.
- Hypotension due to increased intra-abdominal pressure resulting in decreased venous return.
- Bradyarrhythmias during peritoneal or pelvic organ manipulation secondary to vagal stimulation.
- Perforation of the intestines or damage to the abdominal viscera or uncontrolled bleeding (require conversion to a laparotomy).
- Regurgitation.
- Pneumothorax.
- Gas embolism.

CANCER SURGERY

Patients presenting for gynaecological cancer surgery may be elderly, frail, anaemic and cachexic. Ovarian cancers may be present as a large intra-abdominal mass associated with ascites, aortocaval compression or pleural effusion.

Intraoperative considerations

- General anaesthesia using muscle relaxants with or without epidural analgesia is appropriate. Epidural analgesia ensures adequate postoperative pain relief.
- Rapid sequence induction is indicated if the intra-abdominal pressure is increased because of a mass, ascites or both.
- In patients with massive ascites, induction of anaesthesia may be associated with severe hypotension. A surgeon should be ready to perform immediate laparotomy to relieve the intra-abdominal pressure.

OPHTHALMIC SURGERY

The patients can be from the extremes of the age range. The commonest procedure in adults is cataract surgery.

ANAESTHESIA

The eye can be anaesthetized easily with local anaesthetic block and many short procedures (such as cataract extraction and lens implant) can be performed under a local block. The choice of anaesthesia depends on the patient's cooperation, length of operation and expected surgical difficulty. One must make sure that the patient can lie supine without moving, coughing or straining before regional anaesthesia is planned. Unexpected movement or strain when the globe is open can lead to vitreous expulsion, injuries or choroidal haemorrhage. General anaesthesia is used for most children, oculoplastic work and surgery on the posterior part of the eye.

Regional anaesthesia

Regional anaesthesia can be performed by retrobulbar, peribulbar, or sub-Tenon's blocks, or by topical anaesthesia of the cornea. Further details of these blocks is beyond the scope of this book.

The risks of complications (seizures and coma) from injection of local anaesthetic into the sheath around the optic nerve with either peribulbar or retrobulbar block mean that monitoring (usually pulse oximetry) should be used and resuscitation equipment should be available.

OPEN EYE OPERATIONS

In perforated eye injuries it is important to prevent sudden increases in intraocular pressure (IOP). Succinylcholine use leads to an increase in IOP and is best avoided in these patients. However, if it has to be given because of a potentially full stomach, use of an intravenous induction agent will attenuate the rise in IOP. Co-induction with an opioid may also help to limit the rise in IOP.

SQUINT SURGERY

Some patients have associated musculoskeletal disorders. The oculo-cardiac reflex produces bradycardia, hypotension or dysrhythmia during manipulation of the intraocular muscles. Prompt treatment includes stopping the manipulation and use of an anticholinergic agent. Postoperative nausea and vomiting is common.

RETINAL SURGERY

General anaesthesia is usually used, and prevention of the oculo-cardiac reflex is important. An intravitreol gas bubble is sometimes used and nitrous oxide should be avoided.

ORTHOPAEDIC SURGERY

The main considerations for patients undergoing orthopaedic surgery are:

- positioning during surgery
- intraoperative blood loss
- postoperative pain
- high incidence of deep vein thrombosis.

Because many of the major orthopaedic procedures such as joint arthroplasty are performed on elderly patients, pre-existing conditions are encountered more often in these patients (see Table 12.2). Thorough assessment is essential. These procedures are often elective and pre-existing conditions should be actively managed to reduce perioperative risk as much as possible.

Fracture and trauma surgery in young healthy patients should not be problematic. However, long bone fractures and fractures of the pelvis can be associated with significant (and often concealed) haemorrhage. Patients must be adequately resuscitated prior to induction of anaesthesia. Hip fracture is common, especially in osteoporotic elderly women. For these patients fracture fixation should not be delayed to manage long-term conditions, but acute medical conditions such as arrhythmia, heart failure or chest infection should be treated first.

TABLE 12.2 Pre-existing conditions in patients for orthopaedic surgery

Advanced age
Ischaemic artery disease
Hypertension
Rheumatoid arthritis
Steroid therapy
Difficulty in opening mouth or extending neck
Arthritic changes and limitations to positioning
Anatomic abnormalities at the site of regional anaesthesia

ANAESTHETIC MANAGEMENT

Regional anaesthesia or a combination of regional anaesthesia
with general anaesthesia is suitable for many elective orthopaedic
operations. The advantages of regional anaesthesia for orthopaedic
surgery are given in Table 12.3. Spinal or epidural anaesthesia must
be performed with care as elderly patients may have difficulty in com-
pensating for a fall in preload or afterload. Regional anaesthesia (or
analgesia) is avoided when there is a risk of compartment syndrome,
for example after surgery on the tibia.

POSITIONING

Hip surgery is usually performed in the lateral position. Pressure
points must be protected and the arms protected from excessive
compression and from stretching of the brachial plexus. Most other
surgery is performed supine. Surgery to the shoulder and humerus
is usually performed in the semi-sitting (or deck-chair) position. The
patient must be raised to this position slowly ensuring that the blood
pressure is adequate to maintain perfusion of the brain. Venous air
embolism is a risk whenever the operative site is above the level of the
heart. The head and neck should be fixed in a neutral position.

TOURNIQUETS

Tourniquets are used when operating below the humerus or on the
knee or lower leg. The tourniquet pressure is kept at 100 mmHg
above the systolic pressure. Before the tourniquet is inflated, the
limb is usually elevated or one of a variety of methods can be used
to squeeze venous blood out. The duration of safe tourniquet inflation is considered to be 1.5 h for the arm and 2–2.5 h for the leg.
Release of the tourniquet can lead to transient systemic metabolic
acidosis due to the release of the products of hypoxic metabolism

---

**TABLE 12.3 Advantages of regional anaesthesia or analgesia for
orthopaedic surgery**

Improved postoperative analgesia
Decreased incidence of nausea and vomiting
Reduced postoperative respiratory depression
Decreased intraoperative blood loss
Reduced incidence of deep vein thrombosis

into the general circulation. This may cause hypotension, which is usually transient. However, intravenous fluids and the use of a vasopressor agent (increments of phenylephrine or ephedrine) may be required to treat hypotension. During surgery, tourniquet pain can manifest as hypertension. Opioids may help, but sometimes the hypertension is resistant to either analgesics or deepening anaesthesia. Tourniquets should not be used on patients with sickle cell disease.

COMPLICATIONS OF ORTHOPAEDIC SURGERY

Fat embolism

The incidence of fat embolism following fractures of a long bone is 5% and the mortality of an embolus is up to 35%. Patients at risk are those with multiple trauma, particularly if fixation involves intramedullary instrumentation or cementing. Clinical signs usually occur within 12–48 h of the injury, and can range from mild dyspnoea to coma. Other signs include tachycardia, hyperthermia, petechiae, retinal fat emboli, urinary fat globules, decreased platelet count, increased ESR and disseminated intravascular coagulation (DIC). The main criteria for diagnosis of fat emboli syndrome are axillary or sub-conjuctival petechiae, hypoxia, central nervous system depression which is disproportionate to the hypoxia, and pulmonary oedema. Treatment is symptomatic.

Deep vein thrombosis and pulmonary embolism

Venous thromboembolism is a major cause of morbidity and mortality after major surgery or trauma to the lower limbs. Prophylactic measures include external pneumatic compression devices, low-molecular weight heparin and oral anticoagulation in high-risk patients. Patients receiving regional anaesthesia for lower limb surgery have a lower incidence of thromboembolic complications.

Methylmethacrylate cement reactions

Insertion of bone cement may be associated with hypotension which has been attributed to absorption of the volatile monomer of methylmethacrylate, embolization of air or marrow contents, or an allergic reaction. Treatment is supportive.

Compartment syndrome

Trauma of the lower leg (or occasionally the upper leg or the arm) can be associated with a rise in the pressure of the tissue compartments that can compress blood vessels and nerves leading to pain and swelling initially, and later to permanent ischaemic damage to nerves and muscles. Treatment is by immediate decompression of the affected compartments (by fasciotomy).

Spinal or epidural haematoma
See section on central neuraxis blockade for the risks and management of this complication.

PLASTIC SURGERY

This speciality includes the management of acute burn injuries (beyond the scope of this book), reconstructive surgery and cosmetic surgery.

CONSIDERATIONS FOR ELECTIVE RECONSTRUCTIVE PLASTIC SURGERY

- The procedures are often prolonged.
- Deformity from scars around the face and neck may cause a difficult airway.
- If surgery is on or near the face the airway must be secured prior to the commencement of surgery; the anaesthetist must be constantly alert for disconnections or accidental extubation.
- Maintain normothermia and avoid injuries to pressure points.
- Blood flow to free grafts may be helped by reducing the haematocrit with plasma volume expanders such as starch solutions.

UROLOGICAL SURGERY

Endoscopic surgery is very common and many patients such as those with recurrent small bladder tumours return for frequent endoscopic cystoscopy and are often elderly. At the other end of the scale some open urological surgery may be very major and invasive. Patients with a degree of renal failure (acute or chronic) are often seen and need appropriate investigation and preparation for anaesthesia and surgery.

IRRIGATION SOLUTIONS

The irrigation solution used during endoscopic surgery should be isotonic, non-haemolytic and non-toxic. It should allow clear visibility with rapid excretion from the body if absorbed. It should be non-conductive. Normal saline and Ringers lactate are not suitable as they conduct electric currents. Glycine 1.5% allows good visibility. It is a non-electrolyte solution and is slightly hypo-osmolar. If absorbed, glycine is metabolized by the liver. If large quantities are absorbed it can cause toxicity (see TURP syndrome, below).

ENDOSCOPIC CYSTOSCOPY

Flexible cystoscopy can be performed with local anaesthesia only. However, general or regional anaesthesia is required for rigid, prolonged or extensive surgery or if the patient is likely to be unco-operative. If regional anaesthesia is planned, a sensory block up to T6 for upper tract (ureter) manipulation and up to T10 for lower tract manipulation is required.

TRANSURETHRAL RESECTION OF PROSTATE (TURP)

Either regional or general anaesthesia can be used for TURP surgery. Regional anaesthesia has the following advantages:

- atonic large bladder and therefore better surgical visualization
- TURP syndrome (see below) is recognized more easily in awake patients
- better haemostasis due to absence of bladder spasm.

During TURP large venous sinuses are opened up during resection and systemic absorption of irrigating fluid is highly likely. It can be minimized by keeping the height of the fluid column to less than 70 cm and by minimizing the opening of venous sinuses (experienced surgeon). One other important complication of TURP or cystoscopy is bladder perforation which is diagnosed as supra-pubic fullness, pain, spasm, hypo- or hypertension, and hypothermia.

TURP syndrome

This is due to excessive absorption of the non-electrolyte solution into the blood. It causes hyponatraemia and fluid overload which can manifest any time intra- or postoperatively. In an awake patient the signs and symptoms are headache, dizziness, confusion, short-ness of breath, nausea and visual disturbance. Later signs include seizures, stupor and cardiovascular collapse. In a patient under general anaesthesia, TURP syndrome manifests as fluctuations in blood pressure, bradycardia, wide QRS complex, elevated ST segments and ventricular tachycardia.

The treatment of TURP syndrome is:

- inform surgeon and stop irrigation
- give diuretics and restrict i.v. fluids
- give normal saline if serum sodium is more than 120 mmol/litre
- give hypertonic saline if serum sodium is less than 120 mmol/litre. However, frequent estimations of plasma sodium should be made and the hyponatraemia corrected slowly
- arrange admission to a critical care area
- symptomatic treatment with anticonvulsants or sedation.

VASCULAR SURGERY

The management of aortic surgery is beyond the scope of this book and only peripheral vascular surgery will be considered in this chapter.

VARICOSE VEIN SURGERY

Varicose vein surgery is often performed as a day case procedure. Patients for bilateral surgery or recurrent varicose vein surgery may be inpatients. Excessive bleeding is only rarely a problem and routine surgery is not particularly painful. Local anaesthesia can be injected into a groin incision, if one has been made. Beware of accidental femoral nerve block leading to reduced mobility in daycase patients.

PERIPHERAL VASCULAR SURGERY

Patients with peripheral vascular disease have an increased incidence of co-existing medical problems such as diabetes, ischaemic heart disease and chronic obstructive pulmonary disease.

Preoperative considerations

- A full cardiac evaluation, including assessment of exercise tolerance.
- Diabetes should be controlled.
- Optimize pulmonary function.
- Patients may be anticoagulated (preventing the use of central neuraxis or regional blockade).

Intraoperative considerations

- Consider invasive monitoring (CVP line, arterial line) in patients with myocardial dysfunction, exercise limitation or multiple medical problems.
- Careful estimation of fluid status, electrolyte balance and blood loss.
- Careful maintenance of body temperature and assessment of organ perfusion (use a urinary catheter).
- Regional analgesia blocks the stress response, reduces hyper-coagulability, improves graft blood flow and provides postoperative pain relief. However, it may not be tolerated for prolonged procedures.
- Anticoagulation may be used intraoperatively providing 30 min has elapsed since central neuraxis blockade was performed.
- General anaesthesia using a balanced technique with regional block is appropriate for most cases.

Postoperative considerations

- Depending on preoperative status and the operation performed, monitor in a High Dependency Unit.
- Epidural analgesia or regional block to ensure good perfusion of graft.
- Regular assessment of graft function.

EMERGENCY PERIPHERAL VASCULAR SURGERY

This is indicated for severe limb ischaemia resulting from sudden arterial occlusion. Surgical procedures range from simple balloon embolectomy to complex bypass graft surgery. Patients are often anticoagulated preoperatively and regional block will be contra-indicated. However, simple embolectomy in elderly or frail patients can usually be performed with local anaesthesia only.

Perioperative considerations include:

- Co-existing illnesses
- Hyperkalaemia due to limb ischaemia
- Metabolic acidosis
- Tissue damage and myoglobinaemia
- Risk of developing circulatory shock and renal failure.

CHAPTER 13

ANAESTHESIA FOR SPECIAL SITUATIONS

ANAESTHESIA FOR DAY CASE SURGERY

Procedures which are associated with low intensity postoperative care, and can be managed at home and are without serious complications are suitable for day case surgery. Day case surgery is increasingly popular with patients and healthcare organizations and the range of procedures considered suitable is increasing. Patients not usually considered suitable for day case surgery are listed in Table 13.1.

Most day case surgery units have a standardised system of preoperative assessment run by nurses and theatre practitioners. The patient is given instructions about:

- time of arrival, operation and discharge
- preoperative starvation
- preoperative medication
- clear instructions about postoperative pain relief.

ANAESTHETIC MANAGEMENT

The anaesthetic management is broadly similar to that used elsewhere. General anaesthesia is usually used but drugs with a prolonged action or side-effects, for example long-acting opioids, are usually avoided. General anaesthesia is frequently combined with local anaesthetic infiltration or nerve blocks. There is no evidence that local or regional anaesthesia has any particular benefit over general anaesthesia in the day case surgery setting. However, local anaesthetic blocks are often combined with a general anaesthetic for perioperative pain relief and to reduce the amount of anaesthetic needed. Spinal anaesthesia can be used for lower abdominal, perineum or pelvic surgery. Post-dural puncture headaches and

---

TABLE 13.1 Patients inappropriate for day case surgery

- Premature infants
- Anticipated major blood loss
- ASA 3 patients if poorly controlled
- ASA 4 or 5 patients
- Surgery requiring prolonged postoperative monitoring
- Surgery requiring long-term opioids for pain relief
- Morbid obesity
- Current or recent URTI
- No responsible adult to escort home, and care for the patient
- Uncooperative or unreliable patient

urinary retention may require hospital admission. Nerve blocks such as axillary nerve block for hand surgery or ilioinguinal nerve block for inguinal hernia repair are commonly used. Anti-emetic medication is usually given, especially for high-risk procedures such as gynaecological surgery. Non-opioid analgesics such as paracetamol and NSAIDs and weak opioids such as dihydrocodeine are given to the patient to take home.

DISCHARGE

The following should be confirmed before the patient is considered fit for discharge:

- no bleeding from the operation site
- stable vital signs
- able to retain oral fluids
- adequate pain control
- able to walk
- able to pass urine
- absence of debilitating nausea or vomiting.

The failed discharge or readmission rate to day case surgery units is about 1%, although this will vary according to the case-mix. The main factors are nausea and vomiting, pain and bleeding.

ANAESTHESIA FOR THE ELDERLY

PHYSIOLOGICAL CHANGES

Cardiovascular system

Cardiovascular disease is common in the elderly but may be symptomless. Atherosclerosis widens the pulse pressure leading to an increase in systolic arterial pressure; a systolic arterial pressure of up to 180 mmHg may be normal. Ventricular muscle hypertrophy decreases ventricular compliance and there is an increased reliance on filling pressure (preload) to maintain an adequate cardiac output. Heart valves may be fibrosed or calcified. There is an increased incidence of postural hypotension due to impaired autonomic nervous system reflexes and impaired compensation for changes in fluid and blood volume or hypotensive effects of sedatives and anaesthetics.

Respiratory system

Reduced elasticity of the lung tissue increases closing volume, leading to alveolar closure during normal tidal volume respiration. The dead space is increased. Impaired cough reflexes and a reduction in forced vital capacity allow secretions to be retained, and there is an increased incidence of pneumonia.

Central nervous system

Anaesthetic requirements (MAC) are reduced and there is an increased sensitivity to sedative drugs and narcotics.

Other changes

- Reduced renal and hepatic blood flow.
- Reduced body muscle mass.
- Reduced heat production and increased incidence of perioperative hypothermia.
- Altered drug distribution, reduced clearance of drugs.

ANAESTHETIC CONSIDERATIONS

- Elderly people are at increased risk of perioperative morbidity and mortality.
- Many elderly people are hard of hearing and communication can be difficult.
- Poor mobility.
- More sensitive to sedatives and narcotics.
- Because drug clearance is reduced, repeated doses should be administered less frequently.
- Urinary retention or incontinence is common in the perioperative period.
- Increased incidence of postoperative confusion.

OBESITY

Patients with a body mass index (BMI = body weight [kg] $\div$ height^2 [m^2]) greater than 30 are classified as obese. Those with a body mass index of >35 are classified as morbidly obese. Normal body mass index is around 24. Even a modest increase in BMI (~28) is associated with an increased incidence of perioperative complications.

ANATOMIC FEATURES OF THE UPPER AIRWAY IN OBESE PATIENTS

- Short, thick neck
- Redundant pharyngeal and palatal soft tissue

- Large tongue
- Potentially difficult airway and difficult intubation.

PATHOPHYSIOLOGICAL CHANGES

Pathophysiological changes are detailed in Table 13.2.
These physiological changes may lead to:

- hypercarbia
- hypoxaemia
- polycythaemia
- pulmonary hypertension
- congestive heart failure
- sleep apnoea syndrome.

DRUG HANDLING

Fat soluble drugs such as the intravenous induction agents have an increased volume of distribution and a longer elimination half-life. Induction doses are usually calculated on the basis of ideal (lean) rather than actual body weight.

TABLE 13.2 Physiological changes in obesity

Respiratory system

Increased oxygen consumption and carbon dioxide production
Increased work of breathing
Decreased chest wall compliance
Decreased functional residual capacity (FRC) leading to alveolar closure during normal tidal exchange

Cardiovascular system

Increased cardiac output
Increased total blood volume
Systemic hypertension
Pulmonary hypertension secondary to hypoxia
Ventricular hypertrophy and impaired ventricular function

Gastrointestinal system

Increased incidence of hiatus hernia
Increased gastric fluid volume and acidity
Increased intra-abdominal pressure
Gastro-oesophageal reflux

PREOPERATIVE EVALUATION

In addition to routine examination and investigations, echocardiography, arterial blood gases, pulmonary function tests and blood glucose levels may be required in cases of morbid obesity. Premedication with drugs to decrease gastric acidity (H_2 antagonists or proton pump inhibitors) should be considered.

ANAESTHETIC MANAGEMENT

- A tracheal tube provides the most satisfactory means for maintenance of the airway.
- For massively obese patients consider awake tracheal intubation.
- Adequate preoxygenation is essential before induction of anaesthesia because reduced functional residual capacity (especially when positioned supine) and increased oxygen consumption leads to rapid desaturation during apnoea.
- After calculating the dose of induction agent from the ideal body weight, titrate the actual amount given according to the patient's need.
- Use inhalational agents which are least fat soluble.
- Long-acting sedatives, hypnotics and opioids should be used with caution in those at risk of sleep apnoea.

Regional anaesthesia may be preferable because of cardiovascular complications but may be difficult because of indistinct landmarks. Spinal anaesthesia can be used for lower abdominal and extremity surgery. It is usually easier to insert a spinal needle in the sitting position in obese patients.

POSTOPERATIVE CARE

Morbidly obese patients should be managed in a high dependency area postoperatively. They should be recovered in a semi-sitting position and encouraged to sit up and stand as quickly as possible. Because of the increased risk of respiratory depression and sleep apnoea, these patients should be kept in the high dependency area for 2–3 days until the requirement for postoperative analgesia is reduced.

EMERGENCY SURGERY

Common emergency operations include:

- **General surgery**
  Appendicectomy
  Ischiorectal and other abscesses
  Laparotomy for obstruction
  Trauma (blunt or penetrating)
  Strangulated hernia
  Gastrointestinal haemorrhage
- **Vascular surgery**
  Ruptured abdominal aortic aneurysm
- **Gynaecology**
  Evacuation of retained products of conception
  Laparoscopy/laparatomy for ectopic pregnancy or ovarian cyst
- **Orthopaedics**
  Open fracture
  Multiple trauma.

Each of these specialities (and indeed procedures) have some unique features, however this chapter is concerned with the basic principles of anaesthetic management of emergency surgery. Emergencies can be divided into groups using the degree of urgency for the operation. The classification most commonly used is the Confidential Enquiry into Perioperative Deaths (CEPOD) description. CEPOD 1 (or emergency) cases require operations within 1 h for life or limb threatening conditions, for example a ruptured abdominal aortic aneurysm. CEPOD 2 (or urgent) cases require operations within 24 h, for example intestinal obstruction or major fractures. Some CEPOD 1 cases may have only limited assessment and resuscitation performed; often resuscitation occurs at the same time as anaesthesia (or can not take place until after surgery has commenced – major ongoing haemorrhage from penetrating trauma, for example). However, many CEPOD 1 cases and CEPOD 2 cases can be fully resuscitated prior to anaesthesia. CEPOD 2 cases can be fully assessed and can often be delayed for a short time to allow further investigations and management of pre-existing illness.

Emergency cases are performed at any time of the day, but less urgent cases should not be performed after midnight. Trainee anaesthetists should be wary of caring for sick patients by themselves. It is imperative to ensure you do not start a case beyond your skills and capabilities, especially at night when help may not be immediately available in the theatre suite. The care these patients receive in terms of the seniority of personnel, monitoring, intraoperative care and postoperative facilities must be equal to that used for elective cases and must not suffer because of the time of day (or night) that the cases are undertaken.

PREOPERATIVE ASSESSMENT

Fluid status

Blood loss from the gastrointestinal tract may be due to ulcers, neoplasms, oesophageal varices or haemorrhoids. Clear fluid loss may be due to:

● vomiting
● diarrhoea
● peritonitis – significant third space loss into the lumen of the bowel or interstitium
● fever.

Physical signs of hypovolaemia should be looked for (Table 13.3).

Patients who may have lost blood or fluids must have the deficits replaced preoperatively (see Chapter 11). There is some evidence that patients with a ruptured abdominal aortic aneurysm or bleeding secondary to penetrating trauma are not helped by vigorous fluid resuscitation prior to initial surgery to clamp off the bleeding vessel or control the bleeding point. Patients in shock or those with significant co-morbidity should have insertion of a central venous line, assessment of filling pressures and relatively rapid infusion of fluid or blood to restore vital signs to normal before induction of anaesthesia.

METABOLIC DERANGEMENTS

Large gastric losses due to vomiting or nasogastric drainage lead to hypochloraemic metabolic alkalosis. Large diarrhoeal losses or

---

TABLE 13.3 Signs of hypovolaemia

Postural hypotension
Dry mucous membranes
Skin mottling
Decreased skin turgor
Decreased capillary refill
Oliguria
Tachycardia and hypotension in severe cases

septicaemia can cause metabolic acidosis. Sepsis can also produce coagulopathy from disseminated intravascular coagulation.

REFLUX PROPHYLAXIS

Premedication with an H_2 antagonist or proton pump inhibitor and oral non-particulate antacid is recommended in patients at risk of gastro-oesophageal reflux. Prokinetic agents such as metoclopramide are of little benefit and should not be used in cases of bowel obstruction.

ANAESTHESIA

With the exceptions described above anaesthesia should not be induced until the patient is adequately resuscitated including correction of any metabolic disturbances. If the patient remains unstable or sudden deterioration after induction is predicted, an arterial line should be inserted beforehand. However, emergency surgery in a bleeding patient should not be delayed to allow insertion of lines. Patients who are this ill are usually induced in theatre on the operating table to allow the surgeons to gain control of the bleeding as soon as possible after induction of anaesthesia.

Choice of anaesthetic agent

All the commonly used induction agents can be used with care. However, propofol is associated with the greatest fall in blood pressure and thiopental is probably a better alternative. There is some evidence that etomidate is the most cardiovascularly stable of these drugs, although whether this is so in a hypovolaemic patient is unclear. All these agents should be used in smaller doses than in elective surgery. This has to be balanced against the need, when using the rapid sequence induction technique, of choosing a 'sleep' dose and giving all of this and rapidly progressing to giving succinylcholine. Co-induction with a short-acting opioid, such as fentanyl, is thought to be more cardiovascularly stable. However, reductions in the dose of these drugs in shocked patients are also necessary. Any of the currently available maintenance techniques can be used. Again, caution with the quantity of delivered anaesthetic is necessary.

Analgesia

Patients who have lost a large quantity of blood may have a coagulopathy (even if they have received a blood transfusion) and central neuraxis blockade may not be safe until clotting studies have been performed. Intravenous opioids are usually used.

POSTOPERATIVE CARE

Patients with significant co-morbidity, those who were markedly hypovolaemic preoperatively, or remain unstable or on inotropes should be cared for in an HDU or ICU ward. Fluid shifts usually continue postoperatively. Multiple trauma cases, very unstable patients, or those with respiratory complications (for example secondary to elevated intra-abdominal pressure) often require post-operative lung ventilation until their condition improves.

ANAESTHESIA OUTSIDE THE OPERATING SUITE

Anaesthesia may have to be given in locations distant from the operating suite. Common procedures include electroconvulsive therapy (ECT), cardioversion and diagnostic or therapeutic procedures in the radiology department.

GUIDELINES FOR ANAESTHESIA AWAY FROM THE OPERATING THEATRES

- Ensure you are familiar with the orientation and the staffing of the location.
- Ensure that you are familiar with local guidelines regarding supervision, anaesthesia techniques and recovery of the patient.
- An oxygen source should be available for the duration of the procedure.
- A reliable source of suction, and gas scavenging (if inhalational anaesthesia is to be used) should be available.
- The provision of anaesthesia equipment and monitoring should conform to the standards recommended for operating theatres.
- Routine drugs and intravenous fluids should be available.
- Resuscitation drugs available.
- Trained anaesthesia assistant present.
- A self-inflating bag, defibrillator and other equipment to provide effective CPR available.
- A reliable means of communication to other staff.
- Help readily available, if required.

ELECTROCONVULSIVE THERAPY

Anaesthesia is administered in psychiatric units to patients suffering from major affective disorders including severe depression. A grand mal seizure is electrically induced; it consists of a short tonic phase (10–15 seconds) followed by clonic phase which may last for up to a minute.

In physiological terms, ECT can cause brady or tachyarrhythmias, apnoea, hypertension, increased intraocular pressure, increased intragastric pressure and increased ICP. All effects are short lasting and usually self-limiting. However, ECT is contraindicated in patients with intracranial pathology, recent MI and recent cerebrovascular accidents. Care may also be required in pregnancy and long bone fractures.

Preoperative considerations
- Orient yourself with the staff, equipment and procedure.
- Patients may be severely depressed and/or aggressive.
- Pre-existing illnesses (particularly heart problems) should be investigated and their impact minimized.

Anaesthetic considerations
- Pre-oxygenate.
- Minimal monitoring standards are mandatory – these include ECG, NIBP, end-tidal carbon dioxide and pulse oximetry.
- i.v. induction with thiopental (3 mg/kg) or propofol (2 mg/kg) followed by a small dose of suxamethonium (0.5–1.0 mg/kg) and face-mask ventilation is the usual technique. Insertion of a bite-block or oral airway prevents tongue biting during the seizure.
- Patients are placed in the recovery position after the seizure has subsided and breathing has resumed.

CARDIOVERSION

DC cardioversion may be required urgently for patients with SVT or VT and in cardiogenic shock. It is also performed electively for patients with atrial fibrillation. These latter patients will often be anticoagulated.

The DC shock is administered by a cardiologist after the patient has been anaesthetized with an intravenous agent and pre-oxygentated. The choice of agent will depend on the clinical circumstance; for elective procedures propofol is satisfactory.

An oral airway may be inserted, but the anaesthetist will have to release their hold on the face/jaw while the shock is administered. If more than one shock is required, repeat doses of the intravenous agent may be necessary to maintain anaesthesia.

> ⚠ **Following the procedure the heart may be temporarily 'stunned' and the patient's vital signs should be monitored until they have fully recovered.**

RADIOLOGY

During interventional procedures the anaesthetist, along with other staff, will be in the procedure room wearing an X-ray lead gown. The advice of radiology staff in reducing exposure to ionizing radiation should be heeded. During a CT scan the anaesthetist will usually watch the patient from the control room. The room should be arranged to allow the anaesthetist to continuously view the patient, monitor and anaesthetic machine. The patient will move in and out of the scanner and the airway and anaesthetic circuit must be secured to the patient and be able to move freely with them.

Magnetic resonance imaging
Additional precautions:

- Neither patient nor staff should carry with them any ferromagnetic objects such as jewellery, coins, credit cards, watches etc.
- People with pacemakers or implantable defibrillators should not enter the MRI suite. In case of doubt you should consult the MRI radiographer.
- All the anaesthesia and monitoring equipment must be MRI-compatible.

> ⚠ **MRI-compatible equipment may not be 'MRI-safe', as it may be attracted into the magnetic core if it approaches too close. Always familiarize yourself with the instruction manuals for such equipment. Serious injury to staff and patients has occurred when ferromagnetic objects have violently 'leapt' towards the magnet.**

REGIONAL ANAESTHESIA

CENTRAL NEURAXIS BLOCKADE

Regional anaesthesia is the provision of surgical anaesthesia to a part of the body without inducing the loss of consciousness or lack of awareness. Regional anaesthesia techniques can often be used to provide both intraoperative anaesthesia and postoperative analgesia. The patient may remain completely awake and alert, sedative agents may be used to reduce anxiety and dull consciousness, or regional anaesthesia may be combined with general anaesthesia. There are two groups of techniques – central neuraxis blockade (either epidural or subarachnoid blockade) and peripheral nerve blockade. Peripheral nerve blockade is dealt with in Chapter 15.

There are many factors to consider when comparing regional anaesthesia and analgesia with general anaesthesia and a broad statement confirming the superiority of one technique over the other is impossible. However there are certain advantages of each. The main advantages of regional techniques are:

- preservation of consciousness
- preservation of normal respiration
- reduced blood loss
- reduced thrombo-embolic complications
- reduced stress response.

After subarachnoid or epidural anaesthesia, the effect on the respiratory system from paralysis of the intercostal muscles depends on the height of the block. This is usually compensated for by an increase in diaphragmatic movement as a result of reduced tone of the abdominal musculature. Regional techniques are often suitable for patients with respiratory disease. Patients with compromised cardiovascular function may, however, be unsuitable for regional anaesthesia. In particular, patients with a fixed cardiac output state or ischaemic heart disease may not tolerate sudden changes in preload or afterload. While regional techniques are suitable for pelvic, lower limb, upper limb and eye surgery, they are clearly inappropriate when used alone for upper abdominal and thoracic surgery.

Contraindications to central neuraxis blockade include:

- Patient refusal
- Anatomical deformities at the site of injection
- Local or systemic infection
- Anticoagulation therapy or bleeding diathesis

- Hypovolaemia
- Fixed cardiac output states such as aortic stenosis
- Raised intracranial pressure (if central neuraxis blockade is planned).

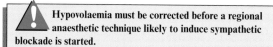

Hypovolaemia must be corrected before a regional anaesthetic technique likely to induce sympathetic blockade is started.

Neurological disease may also be a contraindication although there is no evidence that nerve blockade worsens conditions such as multiple sclerosis. A coagulopathy is a contraindication to central neuraxis blockade. Oral anticoagulants must be stopped, the platelet count should be normal, and low molecular weight heparin (LMWH) should be given at least 12 hours before the block is performed. Postoperative prophylaxis with LMWH may be started after 6 hours, but an in-dwelling catheter should only be removed 12 hours after the last dose of heparin and a further 2 hours should elapse before the next dose is given. There is no evidence that use of non-steroidal anti-inflammatories or aspirin increases the risk of haematoma formation. However, the more potent anti-platelet drugs such as clopidogrel should be treated with the same caution as LMWH.

Possible complications of regional and local anaesthesia are discussed below, but include:

- local anaesthetic toxicity
- hypotension
- urinary retention
- neurological injury
- failure of technique.

GENERAL MANAGEMENT

As with any other anaesthetic technique, regional anaesthesia must only be performed on consented patients, with full resuscitation facilities available.

For all techniques of regional and local anaesthesia full resuscitation facilities must be available.

- Cardiac arrest drugs
- Oxygen supply
- Suction
- Tilting trolley/bed
- Intravenous fluids
- Intubation equipment
- Self-inflating bag or Water's circuit.

Patients about to undergo regional or local anaesthesia should be assessed prior to anaesthesia. The patient should be informed that failure of the regional technique may require progression to general anaesthesia. Preparation should be the same as that of a patient about to undergo general anaesthesia. This includes preoperative starvation. Exceptions to this rule include superficial body surface surgery under local infiltration block and local anaesthesia for ophthalmic surgery.

Safe regional anaesthesia requires a co-operative patient and sedation is usually provided after the block has been performed. However, regional anaesthesia for fracture surgery (for example surgery for a fractured neck of femur) may require analgesia or sedation to position the patient for the regional block. Commonly used agents are midazolam, opioids or ketamine.

When a regional or local technique is combined with general anaesthesia a decision must be taken whether to perform the block before or after induction of general anaesthesia. Some anaesthetists believe that the likelihood of complications such as injection directly into the nerve is less likely in an awake patient; however, there is little evidence to support this belief and many others induce general anaesthesia first.

The central neuraxis blockade techniques are epidural (extra-dural) blockade and subarachnoid (sometimes called spinal) blockade (SAB) (see Figure 14.1). Either of these techniques may be performed with a single bolus dose, intermittent injections via an indwelling catheter or continuous infusion through a catheter. However, placement of a catheter into the subarachnoid space is rarely performed. In general these techniques are suitable to provide anaesthesia for lower limb and pelvic surgery. To provide complete anaesthesia of the upper abdomen and blockade of the nerve supply to the peritoneum (including the vagus nerve) requires a level of blockade likely to produce marked adverse effects. Caesarean section is one of the commonest operations in the lower abdomen (pelvis) performed under central neuraxis blockade and some sensation (but not usually pain) is felt from peritoneal stimulation especially if the uterus is brought out through the abdominal wound.

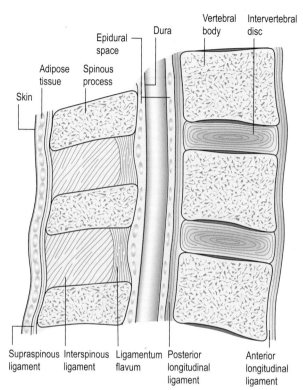

Fig. 14.1 Longitudinal section of structures of spine showing structures to be negotiated when performing an epidural and a spinal (subarachnoid) block.

In subarachnoid blockade the local anaesthetic solution is introduced into the CSF in the low lumbar region after insertion of a needle through the dura and subarachnoid membranes. The technique is similar to diagnostic lumbar puncture. Small quantities of local anaesthetic solution spread rapidly in the CSF producing profound anaesthesia. In epidural blockade the local anaesthetic solution is introduced into the epidural space around the outside of the spinal cord and dura. Usually a catheter is introduced into this space through a needle and local anaesthetic injected via the catheter. The site of injection can be cervical, thoracic, lumbar or caudal. Cervical epidurals are performed in pain management centres for some chronic pain syndromes and are not discussed further here. Caudal injections are usually given via a needle and a catheter is not inserted.

SUBARACHNOID BLOCKADE

The indications for subarachnoid blockade include:

- Transurethral prostatectomy (a block to T10 is required because of innervation of the bladder)
- Hysterectomy
- Caesarean section (block to T6)
- Evacuation of retained products of conception
- Any procedure on the lower limb such as major joint replacement
- Other pelvic and perineal procedures.

Patients for hip and knee replacements are usually elderly and often have concomitant diseases such as respiratory or cardiovascular disease. SAB may be appropriate for these patients providing large changes in cardiac preload and afterload are avoided.

> ⚠ **Intravenous access must be in place before SAB is performed and an infusion of intravenous fluid started. Pre-loading with fluid prior to SAB may reduce the incidence or severity of hypotension.**

POSITION

Lumbar puncture for SAB may be performed in either the sitting (Figure 14.2) or the lateral decubitus position (Figure 14.3). The choice will depend on operator preference, patient comfort and the type of block required. If a saddle block (see below) is required then sitting will be preferable to encourage passage of the local anaesthetic solution to the lowermost parts of the dural sac. However, blockade that must reach the lower thoracic dermatomes will require the patient to lie down soon after the local anaesthetic solution is injected. In the sitting position the patient sits on the edge of the trolley with his/her legs hanging over the side and feet resting on a stool adjusted in height to maintain patient comfort. The patient crosses his/her arms and places them on a pillow on top of the knees. The patient leans forward but more importantly

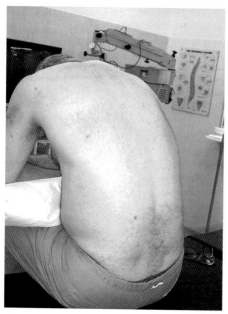

Fig. 14.2 Sitting position used when performing an epidural or spinal block.

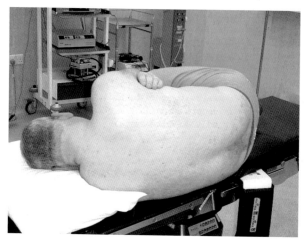

Fig. 14.3 Lateral decubitus position used when performing an epidural or spinal block.

the head and upper thorax are curled forward to open up the spaces between the spinous processes of the lumbar vertebra. An assistant stands in front of the patient to encourage them to adopt the correct position and also to catch the patient should they start to fall.

In the lateral position the patient lies with their back parallel and close to the edge of the trolley. The knees are brought up and the head is curled down and the patient encouraged to adopt a 'curled up in a ball' position. Again an assistant should stand in front of the patient to encourage the correct position.

ANATOMY

A line drawn posteriorly between the iliac crests crosses the midline at the fourth lumbar spinous process or in the third/fourth interspace. The ideal location is the third/fourth interspace but if there is any doubt about the correct level then the space below should be chosen. Inadvertent needle insertion in the second/third interspace may enter the cord or the conus medullaris leading to intense pain and possible permanent damage to the cord.

A full sterile technique is used with drugs drawn from sterile ampoules using a filter needle. The skin is prepared with an antiseptic solution, and sterile drapes placed to isolate non-sterile areas. The skin at the site of needle insertion may be anaesthetized with a small amount of local anaesthetic. Standard practice now is to use a small diameter (usually 25 G) pencil-point needle such as the Sprotte or Whitacre. Use of these needles is associated with the lowest incidence of post-dural puncture headache. Such small calibre needles are usually packaged with a short introducer needle which is used to penetrate the skin and the interspinous ligament. The spinal needle is advanced in the midline, midway between the spinous processes, in a cephalad (towards the head) direction through the interspinous ligament. The needle will pass through the ligamentum flavum and after crossing the epidural space will pierce the dura mater (Figure 14.1). Usually a slight give is felt at this point. Removal of the stylet inside the needle will allow CSF to pass back along the needle and enter the hub. The commonest causes of failure to find the dural sac are poor patient position leading to failure of the spinous processes to open up, or deviation of the needle from the midline.

The needle is held steady while a syringe containing the local anaesthetic solution is attached to the needle hub. Careful aspiration should confirm the free flow of CSF back into the syringe where it will be seen to mix with the local anaesthetic solution. The local anaesthetic solution is then carefully injected – usually over 30–60 seconds. Slow injection allows a hyperbaric solution (see below) to fall under gravity to the dependent parts of the dural sac. Once the injection is complete the needle is removed and a small adhesive plaster is placed over the skin entry site. The patient should then be positioned as required to allow the appropriate block to develop. The blood pressure must be measured every 5 min for at least 20 min as some degree of hypotension (see below) is likely. The upper limit (height) of the block should be assessed by using a cold stimulus (either with ethyl chloride spray or ice) to determine the upper dermatomal level of anaesthesia. Avoid using a potentially skin damaging stimulus such as pin-prick or pinching.

TYPE AND VOLUME OF INJECTATE

Use of hyperbaric (denser than CSF) local anaesthetic solution allows the influence of gravity to partially determine the spread of the local anaesthetic through the CSF. For a block intended to provide anaesthesia for perineal surgery (saddle block) the lower lumbar and sacral dermatomes must be blocked. A small volume of local anaesthetic solution (1–1.5 ml) is used and the patient kept sitting up for the first 3–5 min after the local anaesthetic is injected. For a block intended to block up to the lower thoracic dermatomes a larger volume (3 ml) of local anaesthetic solution is used and the patient is laid down in the supine position as soon as the injection is finished. If the knees are brought up the injectate will spread evenly throughout the lumbar and lower thoracic regions of the cord. If the knees are kept flat the normal lumbar lordosis may prevent adequate spread of the local anaesthetic. The exact upper limit of the block is difficult to predict. It is affected by the volume of injectate, the speed of injection, the height of the patient, the position of the patient during the injection and immediately afterwards, anatomical variations, and pregnancy (a higher than otherwise expected block is common).

The usual agent used for SAB is hyperbaric bupivacaine 0.5%. The bupivacaine is formulated in a 5% glucose solution, increasing its density, which may make it fall under gravity to dependent parts of the subarachnoid space. The usual duration of the block is 2–3 h. The spread of the local anaesthetic and the maximum height of the block are less predictable if a plain (isobaric) solution is used. Small doses of lipid-soluble opioids are often added to the mixture (for example, diamorphine 0.3–0.5 mg) to prolong the duration of analgesia postoperatively.

MANAGEMENT OF COMPLICATIONS

Hypotension

Hypotension is common after SAB because of vasodilatation resulting from the sympathetic block. In general, the higher the block the more widespread the vasodilatation. As well as reducing afterload, preload is reduced. In pregnant patients, pressure of the gravid uterus on the inferior vena cava reduces preload further and pregnant patients should not be permitted to lie supine, but should be tilted to one side. A very high block may directly affect the cardio-accelerator fibres arising from the upper thoracic cord, leading to bradycardia exacerbating the hypotension. Initial treatment is intravenous fluid. Ephedrine may be used prophylactically but is usually used in small boluses (3–6 mg) to treat hypotension not responding to fluids. Atropine may be necessary to correct bradycardia.

Headache

Post-dural puncture headache may be severe and debilitating. Its onset may be up to 5 days after SAB and it may persist for 6 weeks. It is more common in young patients. It is usually worse in the occipital regions and often associated with neck pain, but may be frontal and associated with orbital pain. It is worse on sitting. The incidence is less with the use of small calibre pencil-point needles. Treatment with simple analgesics and encouragement of oral fluids or use of intravenous fluids may be sufficient. Persistent or severe headache should be treated by an epidural 'blood patch' (see Action Plan 25).

Nausea and vomiting

This may occur secondary to hypotension and/or because of unblocked vagal innervation of the abdominal viscera during pelvic and abdominal surgery.

Urinary retention

Retention is common especially if large volumes of fluid are used to treat hypotension.

Other complications

Vasodilatation may lead to hypothermia. Labyrinthine disturbance sixth cranial nerve disturbance, meningitis, transverse myelitis and cauda equina syndrome are all rare sequelae.

EPIDURAL ANAESTHESIA

Epidural anaesthesia usually refers to injection of local anaesthetic solutions (sometimes combined with an opioid) into the
epidural space in the lumbar or low thoracic regions. The upper
or mid-thoracic regions are sometimes used for thoracic or
upper abdominal surgery. In general the best blockade results
from injection near the site of origin of the supplying nerves.
Therefore analgesia for labouring women can be provided by
injection in the low lumbar region, but for midline abdominal surgery injection in the low to mid-thoracic region is best.
Although local anaesthetic solution can be injected through a
needle directly into the epidural space, the usual technique
is to place a catheter into the epidural space and then make
intermittent injections or start a continuous infusion through
the catheter. Only the technique for lumbar epidural catheter
placement and use will be described.

Local anaesthetics in the epidural space can be used to
provide operative anaesthesia although this may be difficult to
achieve in some patients. Epidural analgesia is more commonly
used to provide intraoperative and postoperative analgesia.
Bolus doses are usually used for intraoperative analgesia but
for postoperative use epidural infusions are usually used. A low
concentration of local anaesthetic is often combined with a
small dose of short-acting, lipid-soluble opioid such as fentanyl.
With long-term use regular observations for an extending block,
hypotension, urinary retention and respiratory depression must
be made.

TECHNIQUE FOR EPIDURAL ANAESTHESIA

The epidural catheter is placed through a widebore 'seeker' needle inserted into the epidural space with the patient positioned
in either the sitting or lateral decubitus position (as described
for SAB above). The key to safe performance of this technique
is identification of the epidural space. The seeker needle must
pass through the ligamentum flavum into the epidural space
but not pierce the dural sac. The needles used are called Tuohy
needles (Figure 14.4). They have distance markings every
centimetre, a stylet to assist with skin puncture, and a curved
(Huber) tip which makes dural sac puncture less likely and
assists in positioning the catheter into the epidural space. Post-
dural puncture headache resulting from the passage of a Tuohy

needle through the dura may be very problematic. An incorrectly placed catheter may remain outside the epidural space, or be placed into the large epidural venous plexus, or be inserted under the dura but outside the arachnoid space (subdural), or into the CSF itself.

After positioning the patient in the sitting or lateral decubitus position, the skin is cleaned, sterile drapes placed and a small subcutaneous bleb of local anaesthetic is placed at the site of insertion. The Tuohy needle is inserted with its opening orientated superiorly. As the Tuohy needle is advanced towards the epidural space in the midline it passes through the skin, the supraspinous ligament, the interspinous ligament and then the ligamentum flavum. Once the tip of the needle is in the interspinous ligament, the stylet is removed and a low-friction (loss-of-resistance) syringe containing either air or normal saline is attached. The ligamentum flavum is usually quite tough. As the needle and syringe is advanced attempts to inject the air or saline through the needle are made. In general there is resistance to injection – particularly when the tip of the needle is in the ligamentum flavum. As soon as the tip of the needle

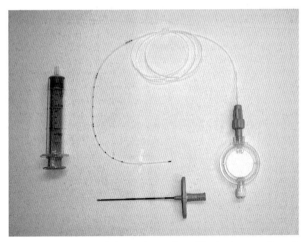

Fig. 14.4 Epidural set including Tuohy needle, epidural catheter and loss-of-resistance syringe.

passes out of the ligamentum flavum and into the epidural space, the resistance to injection suddenly becomes much less. This is known as the 'loss-of-resistance' technique. As the ligamentum flavum is approached the Tuohy needle may either be advanced very slowly with intermittent injections every 2–3 mm, or continuous pressure on the syringe plunger may be applied. The epidural space in the lumbar region is about 5 mm deep. After the epidural space has been identified the needle must not be rotated. The depth markings are noted and the catheter then inserted through the needle. If this proves difficult the whole needle and catheter combination must be removed as one (as removal of the catheter through the needle may result in shearing off of the catheter tip). Initially up to 5 or 6 cm of catheter are inserted through the Tuohy needle. The needle is then removed and the catheter pulled back so that once the depth of tissue between the skin surface and the epidural space has been taken into account there is about 3–5 cm of catheter remaining in the epidural space.

Before the filter and hub are attached to the end of the catheter, it should be inspected for free flow of blood or CSF. It should be remembered that, if used, some of the saline to detect the epidural space may flow back into the catheter. This may be blood-stained if a small blood vessel or the periosteum of bone (for example the lamina) has been damaged. It is important to distinguish between this and the free flow of frank blood or CSF. Careful aspiration of the catheter may suggest placement into the CSF or an epidural vein. However, the lumen of the catheter may collapse under the negative pressure of the aspiration, the vein walls may collapse or the catheter, which has a number of holes along the last few centimetres of its length, may be only partially inside a vein or dural sac, and aspiration may give a false negative result. A test injection of 3 ml of local anaesthetic should be made. This will identify placement of the catheter into the CSF as a much more widespread and profound block will result. However, a test injection will not usually identify placement into an epidural vein. Using a local anaesthetic with addition of 1:200,000 epinephrine will result in an increase in heart rate if injected into an epidural vein. A correctly placed catheter may move during use. A high index of suspicion should be maintained at all times and any signs of extending block or systemic toxicity treated seriously.

TYPE AND VOLUME OF INJECTATE

The spread of local anaesthetic solution through the epidural space is not completely predictable. Important factors are volume of injectate, position of the patient, age and pregnancy. Onset time is reduced by increasing the concentration of the local anaesthetic and by the addition of epinephrine. These factors also determine the duration of action. Although lidocaine is associated with a faster onset, bupivacaine 0.25% or 0.5% are the most commonly used agents because of their longer duration of action. After the test dose has been given, the epidural is usually 'topped-up' with boluses (3–5 ml at a time) of local anaesthetic solution (with or without an opioid) until the block has reached the desired dermatomal level. After this time either further boluses are given (usually intraoperatively) or an infusion of low concentration local anaesthetic agent (usually combined with a low concentration of fentanyl) is started. Regular observations for cardiovascular changes and the height of the block (as for SAB) must be made. After each bolus the blood pressure should be checked every 5 min for at least 20 min.

COMPLICATIONS OF EPIDURAL ANAESTHESIA

- Hypotension
- Nausea and vomiting
- Shivering
- Dural puncture ('dural tap')
- Headache (following dural tap)
- Total spinal anaesthesia (due to large volume of local anaesthetic solution being injected directly into the CSF)
- Subdural block leading to a high, but patchy block
- Toxicity due to intravenous injection or rapid absorption of very large doses
- Epidural haematoma
- Epidural abscess
- Neurological damage either to the cord itself or to nerve roots.

Prolonged blockade, especially if associated with back pain, may be due to an epidural haematoma or abscess. Cord compression may lead to paraplegia if not diagnosed and must be decompressed urgently. Any suggestion of unusual or prolonged blockade must be taken seriously and if unexplained an urgent spinal MRI must be arranged.

CAUDAL (EPIDURAL) ANAESTHESIA

This form of epidural anaesthesia is useful for blocking the lowermost nerve roots from the spinal cord – in particular the sacral and lower lumbar roots. Because it is usually performed as a 'one-off' injection (without placement of a catheter), there is no opportunity to 'top-up' a partial block. Caudal epidurals are not used for intraoperative anaesthesia but good intraoperative and postoperative analgesia for perineal surgery may be obtained. In children, a higher block (to provide analgesia for herniorraphy for example) may be achieved by increasing the volume of the injectate. Widespread sympathetic block is unusual after caudal anaesthesia.

The sacral canal contains the end of the dural sac (usually at the S2 level, but may extend down as far as S4), nerve roots, a venous plexus and fatty tissue. Local anaesthetic is injected into the canal by placing a needle through the sacrococcygeal membrane covering the sacral hiatus (Figure 14.5). The sacral hiatus is formed by a failure of the fifth sacral vertebral lamina to fuse in the midline posteriorly. Sometimes the sacral hiatus extends superiorly due to failure of the fourth vertebra to fuse. Because the upper limit of the hiatus is variable and the lower limit of the dural sac is also variable, it is easy for a needle placed through the sacral hiatus to enter the dural sac. However, the mean distance between the uppermost part of the hiatus and the dural sac in adults is usually 4–5 cm. Careful aspiration must be performed to ensure that CSF cannot be drawn back before injection of a large volume of local anaesthetic for the caudal block.

The patient is placed in the lateral decubitus position with the hips and knees well flexed to expose the skin over the sacral hiatus. A needle (usually a standard 21 G green needle) is inserted through the sacrococcygeal membrane at 45° to the skin until the membrane is pierced. The needle is then aligned to lie parallel to the skin and advanced a further 1–2 cm. Confirmation that the needle is in the sacral canal and not lying subcutaneously comes from 'wiggling' the needle. If it is in the sacral canal its movements will be limited. If the needle is placed in the subcutaneous fat, it will move more easily and injection of local anaesthetic solution will produce a lump just below the skin. Before injection, careful aspiration to prevent accidental intradural injection must be performed. If there is resistance to injection the needle is incorrectly sited and should be replaced.

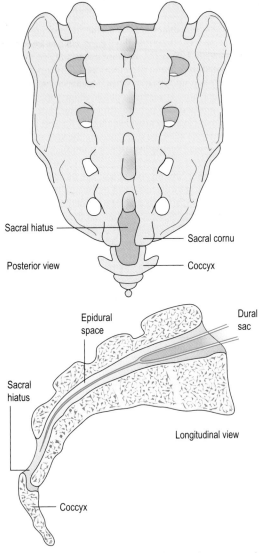

Fig. 14.5 Anatomy of sacrum showing sacral hiatus – the entry route for sacral epidural injections.

INJECTATE

The usual volume of injectate in adults is 20 ml. In children 0.5 ml/kg is used for a low block. If a higher block is required (e.g. hernia repair) up to 1.25 ml/kg may be used. Because of the good absorption from this site, the concentration of local anaesthetic solution may have to be reduced to avoid systemic toxicity.

PERIPHERAL NERVE BLOCKADE

This chapter does not include an exhaustive description of all the major nerve blocks but concentrates on the blocks commonly used:

- axillary nerve block
- femoral nerve block
- sciatic nerve block
- psoas compartment block
- inguinal field block
- ring block
- penile block
- intravenous regional anaesthesia (Bier's Block).

These blocks are usually performed to provide intra- and post-operative analgesia. Although they may be used to provide operative anaesthesia, the block must be complete and last long enough to permit the surgical procedure to be finished. Often general anaesthesia or sedation is combined with these blocks.

GENERAL CONSIDERATIONS

The local anaesthetic agent used for these procedures is usually 0.25 or 0.5% bupivacaine. A large volume of local anaesthetic is used with some of these techniques and the total quantity of agent injected must be calculated to ensure the maximum limits have not been breached (see Chapter 2). L-bupivacaine and ropivacaine are alternatives. Lidocaine may be substituted or used in combination with bupivacaine to increase the speed of onset of the block.

As with any other anaesthetic technique, regional and local anaesthesia must only be performed on consented patients, with full resuscitation facilities available.

 For all techniques of regional and local anaesthesia full resuscitation facilities must be available.

- Cardiac arrest drugs
- Oxygen supply
- Suction
- Tilting trolley/bed
- Intravenous fluids
- Intubation equipment
- Self-inflating bag or Water's circuit.

Intravenous access should always be established before starting a peripheral nerve block. The blocks must be performed carefully to prevent accidental intravascular injection, and to avoid doses of local anaesthetics likely to lead to systemic toxicity following absorption from the site of injection. The contraindications to peripheral nerve blockade include patient refusal, allergy to local anaesthetic agents, local sepsis, and coagulopathy.

TECHNIQUE FOR NERVE LOCATION

Superficial nerves such as inguinal field block, penile block and ring block can be performed using skin landmarks only. However, a technique to correctly identify the position of deeply placed nerves such as the femoral and the sciatic nerve is necessary. When combined with a general anaesthetic these blocks may be performed before or after induction of anaesthesia. A variable output nerve peripheral nerve stimulator (Figure 15.1) and an insulated short-bevelled needle are used to electrically stimulate the nerve. In awake patients the production of paraesthesia along the distribution of the nerve if the injecting needle touches it will also warn of injection too near or into the nerve itself. When performed after induction of anaesthesia, only the nerve stimulator can warn of proximity to the nerve. The aim is to deposit the local anaesthetic solution near to but not in the nerve. Movement in the muscle

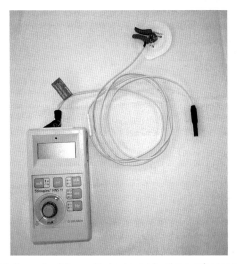

Fig. 15.1 Nerve stimulator used to locate peripheral nerves for nerve block.

groups supplied by the nerve is observed for and when seen the stimulating current is slowly reduced. As the needle tip approaches the nerve the minimum current required to stimulate the nerve falls. If the nerve can be stimulated with a current less than 0.5 mA then the needle tip is within a few millimetres of the nerve and the injection can be performed. Stimulation of the nerve with a current less than 0.2 mA indicates that the needle tip may have entered the nerve itself and that the tip should be withdrawn before injecting. There should be little resistance to injection and the movement in the muscles from the stimulation will cease after injection of less than 1 ml of local anaesthetic solution. Clearly the patient must not have received neuromuscular blocking agents. The use of ultrasound to confirm placement of the needle tip close to nerves is becoming more popular.

AXILLARY BLOCK

ANATOMY

The arm is supplied by the branches of the brachial plexus except for the cutaneous supply to the medial part of the upper limb, which is derived from a branch of the second thoracic intercostal supply called the intercostobrachial nerve. The cords of the brachial plexus enter the axilla and surround the axillary artery and pass distally to form the terminal branches (the median, ulnar and radial nerves).

INDICATION

The axillary approach to the brachial plexus provides analgesia below the elbow joint. Blockade of the radial nerve is not particularly reliable with this technique. Axillary nerve block rarely blocks the musculocutaneous nerve and there is no analgesia on the upper inner aspect of the arm. For analgesia of the upper arm and shoulder region a more proximal approach to the brachial plexus must be used.

TECHNIQUE

- The patient lies supine with the arm abducted and the elbow flexed. The hand may be put behind the head.
- The most medial (proximal) part of the axillary artery is identified in the axilla.

- An insulated needle pierces the skin heading to the apex of the axilla and angled to pass alongside the artery and not pierce it.
- The needle pierces the sheath surrounding the artery and nerves and stimulation results in movement of distal muscles in the arm.
- 30 ml of local anaesthetic solution is injected. Pressure applied just distal to the site of injection may help proximal spread of the solution.

COMPLICATIONS

Accidental puncture of the axillary artery is common. However, if this is managed by firm pressure it should not cause a problem. Some authors advocate deliberate puncture of the artery so that local anaesthetic solution can be injected 'behind' the artery to block the radial nerve.

FEMORAL NERVE BLOCK

ANATOMY

The femoral nerve is derived from the second, third and fourth lumbar roots. It provides a cutaneous supply to the anterior thigh, the knee extensor muscles, and the hip and knee joints. The femoral nerve terminates in the saphenous nerve, which supplies the medial border of the lower leg and foot. It enters the thigh below the inguinal ligament just lateral to the femoral artery (see Figure 15.2). The obturator nerve and the lateral cutaneous nerve of the thigh are formed from the lumbar plexus above the inguinal ligament and supply the upper part of the lower limb and need to be blocked to provide complete analgesia. This may be achieved by using the three-in-one technique when pressure applied just distal to the injection site for femoral nerve block helps local anaesthetic solution pass proximally up the sheath surrounding the femoral nerve and block these other nerves.

INDICATION

Femoral nerve block is used for surgery on the hip, the knee (usually combined with sciatic nerve block), and for analgesia following a fractured femur.

TECHNIQUE

- With the patient lying supine, the inguinal ligament and femoral artery are identified.
- An insulated needle is inserted parallel and 1–2 cm lateral to the artery pointing in a slightly cephalad direction.
- Movement of the patella due to contraction of the quadriceps muscle groups indicates that the needle is close to the femoral nerve. Movement of the sartorius nerve (due to direct stimulation) is inadequate.
- 20 ml of local anaesthetic solution is injected.

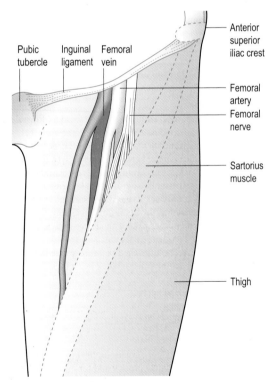

Fig. 15.2 Structures close to femoral nerve in the groin.

COMPLICATIONS

Accidental puncture of the femoral artery.

SCIATIC NERVE BLOCK

ANATOMY

The sciatic nerve is formed from the roots of L4, L5 and S1–S4. It supplies the back of the upper leg, most of the lower leg and most of the foot. The nerve passes through the great sciatic foramen and descends in the posterior part of the thigh before it divides into the tibial and common peroneal nerves. A number of approaches to the sciatic nerve are described. The easiest is the Raj approach as the patient is supine and the surface markings are usually easy to identify.

INDICATION

Operations on the knee or below.

TECHNIQUE

- The patient lies supine.
- The leg is held by an assistant with both the hip and knee flexed at 90°.
- A needle is inserted mid-way between the ischial tuberosity and the greater trochanter, perpendicular to the skin (see Figure 15.3).
- If the needle hits bone (the femur) the needle should be redirected more medially.
- Electrical stimulation when the nerve is approached results in plantar or dorsiflexion of the foot.
- 30 ml of local anaesthetic solution should be injected.

COMPLICATIONS

Complications are very rare.

PSOAS COMPARTMENT BLOCK

ANATOMY

The proximal part of the nerves derived from the L2–L4 roots pass through the substance of the psoas muscle. An injection of a large volume of local anaesthetic solution into the psoas

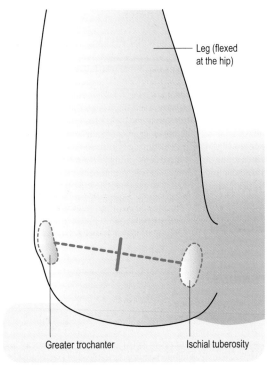

Fig. 15.3 Anatomy of sciatic nerve block. Skin surface landmarks for posterior (Raj) approach to the sciatic nerve block. The leg is flexed at the hip and the knee.

compartment (anterior to the transverse process of L3) will achieve the same result as the 3-in-1 block of the femoral nerve.

INDICATION

Otherwise known as the lumbar plexus block, this is a useful technique for hip fracture surgery.

TECHNIQUE

- The patient is placed in the lateral position and the spinous process of the third lumbar vertebra is identified.

- A long needle is inserted perpendicular to the skin, 3–4 cm lateral to the upper border of the spinous process to strike the transverse process. If bone is not identified the needle should be advanced in a more cephalad direction.
- The needle is 'walked off' the superior edge of the transverse process and then advanced another 2–3 cm until a 'give' is felt.
- Alternatively an insulated needle can be used in the non-paralysed patient and movement in the quadriceps muscle in response to electrical stimulation is elicited.
- 30 ml of local anaesthetic is injected after careful aspiration for blood and CSF.

> ⚠ **Care must be taken to prevent passing the needle towards the midline and entering the epidural or subarachnoid spaces.**

COMPLICATIONS

- Epidural and subarachnoid injection.
- Damage to the kidney.

INGUINAL FIELD BLOCK

ANATOMY

The nerve supply to the skin and tissues in the inguinal region is derived from the subcostal nerve (T12), the iliohypogastric and the ilioinguinal nerves (L1), the genital branch of the genitofemoral nerve (L1 and L2) and a supply crossing from the opposite side. Inguinal field block involves blockage of all these nerves (see Figure 15.4).

INDICATION

This technique is useful for intra- and postoperative analgesia for inguinal hernia surgery. With care and additional infiltration by the surgeon – particularly along the line of incision and of the peritoneal sac – this technique can be used as the sole form of anaesthesia if necessary.

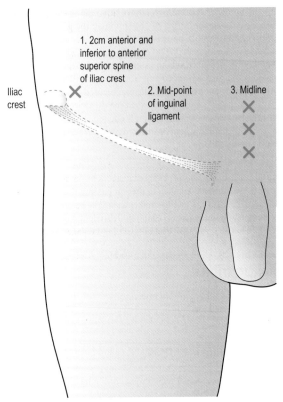

Fig. 15.4 Skin surface landmarks for ilioinguinal block – three injection points.

TECHNIQUE

- The ilioinguinal and the iliohypogastric are blocked by injection 2 cm medial and inferior to the anterior superior iliac crest. The needle is felt to pop as it goes through the aponeurosis of the external oblique muscle.
- 5 ml of local anaesthetic solution is injected, moving the needle around after every 2 ml of injection to ensure that the tissue space is filled with local anaesthetic. Another 5 ml of local anaesthetic solution should also be injected deep to the internal oblique layer.

- 5 ml is injected below the external oblique muscle layer at the midpoint of the inguinal ligament to block the genital branch of the genitofemoral nerve.
- A further 5 ml injection is used to raise a subcutaneous weal in the skin just above the pubic symphysis in the midline to block the nerve supply from the other side.

RING OR DIGITAL NERVE BLOCK

ANATOMY

Each digit is supplied by two nerves on either side. One pair is closer to the palmar surface and the other is more dorsal.

> ⚠️ **Because the blood supply is dependent on an end-artery, vasoconstrictors must not be added to the local anaesthetic solution.**

INDICATION

Operative or postoperative analgesia of a digit.

TECHNIQUE

- A needle is inserted through the skin at the base of the digit from the dorsal side.
- 2–3 ml of local anaesthetic is injected on each side.
- If anaesthesia at the base of the digit is required, the injection can be performed either side of the metacarpal/metatarsal.

PENILE BLOCK

ANATOMY

The nerve supply to the penis is predominantly derived from dorsal nerves of the penis, which are branches of the internal pudendal nerves. They arise from under the pubic symphysis and pass either side of the midline to the base of the penis. An additional supply from scrotal branches of the perineal nerves innervates the ventral surface of the penis.

> ⚠ **Vasoconstrictors must not be added to the local anaesthetic solution as the arterial supply to the penis is an end artery.**

INDICATION

Penile block is a useful technique for intra- and postoperative analgesia for circumcision.

TECHNIQUE

- 5–10 ml of local anaesthetic is injected in the midline between the base of the penis and the pubic symphysis at a depth of about 2 cm.
- Subcutaneous infiltration between the base of the penis and between the penis and the scrotum.

INTRAVENOUS REGIONAL ANAESTHESIA (IVRA)

ANATOMY

A large volume of a low concentration of local anaesthetic solution is injected intravenously into an exsanguinated forearm. Systemic toxicity is prevented by use of a tourniquet. The technique should not be used if the patient has Raynaud's disease or sickle-cell disease.

INDICATION

IVRA is used to provide analgesia for manipulation of a displaced fracture of the forearm bones. It can also be used for intraoperative anaesthesia, for example for carpal tunnel decompression. Performed correctly, it is a simple, safe and effective block. Onset of analgesia is rapid, recovery is quick and the patient can be discharged home shortly afterwards.

TECHNIQUE

- A cannula is inserted into both hands.
- The limb should be exsanguinated by elevation.
- The upper part of a double-cuffed tourniquet is inflated to 100 mmHg above systolic pressure.
- 40 ml of local anaesthetic agent (prilocaine 0.5%) is injected. The tourniquet must remain inflated for at least 20 min after injection to allow diffusion of the agent into the tissues of the arm.
- Tourniquet pain can be reduced by use of the double cuff. After onset of the block the skin and tissues underneath the lower cuff will be anaesthetized and the lower cuff can be inflated, after which the upper cuff can be deflated.
- At the end of the procedure the tourniquet is released and the patient observed for signs of systemic toxicity.

> ⚠ **The tourniquet should not be released for at least 20 min after injection of the local anaesthetic to allow the drug to diffuse into the tissues, even if the surgery is finished before this.**

OTHER ASPECTS OF ANAESTHESIA

POSTOPERATIVE CARE

After anaesthesia – general or regional – patients are admitted to a Recovery Ward (or Post Anaesthesia Care Unit – PACU). In these the ratio of nursing staff to patient is usually 1 to 1, or 1 to 2 for conscious patients. The priorities after general anaesthesia are maintenance of a patent airway, adequate ventilation and oxygen therapy. All patients require regular monitoring of heart rate, peripheral blood saturation and blood pressure. Intravenous fluids may be needed and fluid balance including urine output and loss in surgical drains is recorded.

Patients recall pain and nausea and vomiting as the most distressing after-effects of anaesthesia and surgery. Ensuring patient comfort with adequate pain relief, treatment of postoperative nausea and vomiting (PONV), and treatment of hypothermia is essential.

Failure to recover consciousness after general anaesthesia is dealt with in Action Plan 11.

AIRWAY MAINTENANCE

In the recovery period partial airway obstruction may contribute to hypoventilation. In the unconscious patient the airway should be cleared of blood and oral secretions and the mandible should be displaced anteriorly to lift the tongue forward and away from the posterior pharyngeal wall. Maintenance of a clear airway may be easier if the patient is placed in the lateral position. An oral airway may also help although it may cause gagging and coughing as the patient becomes more conscious. A nasal airway may be better tolerated although there is a risk of causing haemorrhage from the nasal mucosa. Laryngeal mask airways may be left in place for an experienced nurse to remove when the patient is awake. It is not acceptable to leave a non-anaesthetist to care for a patient with a tracheal tube in place (except in the ICU environment). Tracheostomy tubes are usually well tolerated and remain in place postoperatively.

Laryngospasm may occur during emergence from anaesthesia and is dealt with in Action Plan 20.

OXYGEN THERAPY

All patients who have received a general anaesthetic should receive postoperative supplemental oxygen therapy for at least 10 min. This may have to be continued if there are complications after anaesthesia or pulse oximetry demonstrates a failure to adequately oxygenate peripheral blood.

> ⚠️ **Patients who may be sedated for prolonged periods, for example by the use of opioids, should receive supplemental oxygen.**

All general anaesthetic techniques have some effect on respiratory function. Possible factors include:

- reduction in functional residual capacity leading to postoperative atelectasis
- nitrous oxide use is associated with a short period of hypoxia secondary to excretion of nitrous oxide from the lungs (see Chapter 2)
- respiratory drive may be depressed by the residual effects of general anaesthetic agents
- opioid analgesics
- residual neuromuscular blockade.

Postoperative hypoxaemia has been shown to occur particularly at night and may continue for 2–3 days. It is assumed that such hypoxaemia is detrimental and may be a cause of poor wound healing, contribute to the stress response and lead to myocardial ischaemia and infarction.

VARIABLE PERFORMANCE DEVICES

Oxygen therapy may be supplied in several forms by simple variable performance devices:

- Hudson mask
- MC mask
- Nasal cannulae (nasal specs).

These devices increase the inspired concentration of oxygen in the inspired gases by a variable amount. The actual increase depends on the oxygen flow rate, respiratory frequency, tidal volume, length of pause between inspiration and expiration, deadspace of the mask, and the tightness of fit of the mask. Because these factors vary so much from patient to patient the actual oxygen concentration in inspired gas is difficult to predict. Oxygen at 4 L/min via a mask or 2 L/min via nasal specs will usually increase the oxygen concentration in inspired gases to about 30–40%. Higher flows may be unpleasant and lead to the patient removing the oxygen therapy device.

FIXED PERFORMANCE DEVICES

If it is important to administer a known concentration of oxygen to the patient (to help in the interpretation of blood gases results or in some patients with chronic airflow obstruction and chronic hypercapnia who have lost sensitivity to carbon dioxide) a fixed performance device such as the Ventimask should be used. These masks use a Venturi device to entrain a known concentration of air with oxygen to give a predictable increase in the inspired concentration of oxygen applicable to most patients. In addition, the total gas flow rate (oxygen and air) is in excess of the peak inspiratory flow rate of most patients. These masks are available in a number of concentrations – 24%, 28%, 35% and 60%.

In patients with shock, myocardial ischaemia, respiratory failure or after trauma it is important to maximize the inspired concentration of oxygen. 100% oxygen cannot be achieved with these devices (a tightly fitting face-mask or tracheal intubation combined with a non-rebreathing circuit is usually required for this), but a face-mask with an attached reservoir bag should be used and an oxygen flow rate of 15 L/min. This will provide an inspired oxygen concentration greater than 60% for most patients.

CARDIOVASCULAR SYSTEM

Pulse rate and blood pressure are monitored during recovery from anaesthesia and to detect inadequate fluid replacement or on-going bleeding. The management of hypertension and hypotension are dealt with in Action Plans 13 and 14 respectively.

If the patient is catheterized, the urine output should be monitored hourly. A poor urine output is often a sign of hypovolaemia. Oliguria is dealt with in Action Plan 24.

FLUID MANAGEMENT

Patients undergoing minor surgery will either not have had intravenous fluids intraoperatively or, if they did, can stop these in the recovery ward. Some patients require maintenance fluids postoperatively:

● continued nil-by-mouth regime (e.g. after abdominal surgery and likely paralytic ileus)
● high likelihood of PONV
● reduced conscious level.

Others may require fluids postoperatively to replace on-going losses such as:

- postoperative bleeding (e.g. major joint replacement surgery, TURP)
- entero-cutaneous fistula
- major trauma cases.

For these patients the choice of fluids and rate of administration will depend on the normal maintenance requirements and an estimate of likely losses. The types of fluid available are dealt with elsewhere.

TEMPERATURE CONTROL

Core temperature should be measured on arrival in recovery. Many patients cool after surgery finishes as forced warm air blankets and surgical drapes are removed.

SHIVERING

Postoperative shivering in normothermic patients may be unpleasant for the patient and be associated with increased metabolic requirements. It can be treated with small doses (25 mg) of intravenous pethidine.

HYPOTHERMIA

See Action Plan 16.

PONV

See Action Plan 27.

SORE THROAT AND HOARSENESS

Sore throat is a common complication of anaesthesia. It may be due to trauma to the upper airway from a tracheal tube or the process of tracheal intubation or extubation. Sore throat may also occur after use of a laryngeal mask airway or mask anaesthesia. Hoarseness after tracheal intubation is usually short-lived and if it persists for more than 24 h should be assessed by an ENT surgeon. Laryngeal, arytenoid or vocal cord damage may have occurred and may require treatment.

POSTOPERATIVE PAIN RELIEF

The available analgesic agents are discussed in the pharmacology section.

Postoperative pain relief starts with a discussion with the patient as part of the preoperative assessment of likely pain and the choice of analgesic techniques and drugs. Analgesia will nearly always be given intraoperatively and should be planned to continue into the postoperative period. In the recovery ward (and afterwards) pain should be assessed – for example by asking the patient to grade the pain on a 10-point scale, where 0 is 'no pain' and 10 is 'the worst pain imaginable'.

Regional anaesthetic techniques will usually last into the postoperative period. Some techniques such as major nerve blocks like femoral/sciatic nerve block will provide analgesia for up to 36 h.

> ⚠ **Use of local anaesthetic alone in the subarachnoid space is associated with a rapid return of sensation (and pain!). Plan to give other analgesia before the spinal wears off.**

The intraoperative use of nitrous oxide or short-acting opioids alone will not provide postoperative analgesia. Analgesics that can be used intraoperatively that will provide postoperative pain relief include:

- Simple analgesics (paracetamol)
- NSAIDs and COX 2 inhibitors
- Long-acting opioids (e.g. morphine)
- Local anaesthetic nerve blocks, epidural analgesia
- Subarachnoid local anaesthetic combined with a long-acting, intrathecal opioid (e.g. diamorphine).

These agents are used in a graduated manner – paracetamol for surgery associated with mild pain only, the addition of an NSAID for slightly more painful surgery, and long-acting opioids for more painful surgery or when pain is expected to persist. The side-effects of opioids preclude their use for mild pain only. The use of local anaesthetic blocks may make opioids unnecessary or substantially reduce the dose and, hopefully, the side-effects.

PARENTERAL OPIOIDS

For many types of surgery parenteral opioids are required postopertively, and morphine is the commonest drug used.

The patient will usually be 'loaded' intraoperatively. However, as dose requirements can vary by as much as 10-fold between patients, many patients may not be pain-free on emergence. In the recovery ward small boluses of morphine (2–5 mg) are given, with close monitoring for sedation and depression of ventilation. If not already given, prophylactic anti-emetics are administered (see PONV Action Plan 27).

> ⚠ **Facilities for resuscitation and personnel trained in airway management must be available whenever parenteral opioids are administered.**

Intravenous morphine may start to work within 5–10 min. An alternative agent may be added to the regime – such as paracetamol or an NSAID if not already given, or a different opioid such as tramadol. If the requirement for morphine is likely to continue, the commonest technique for administration is patient-controlled analgesia (PCA).

PATIENT-CONTROLLED ANALGESIA

The patient activates a pre-filled pump administering themselves a small bolus (usually 1 mg) of morphine intravenously. After each injection the pump is 'locked out' for 5 min, before it will accept instructions from the patient to administer another bolus. The fact that the patient activates the pump is a safety feature in that if the patient becomes drowsy they can't administer any more morphine to themselves. PCA appears to be safe providing a background infusion is not used. If pain relief is not effective the size of the bolus can be increased.

Patients whose morphine requirements are not great may manage with intermittent subcutaneous injections. There is no justification for the intramuscular route. Some patients may not be able to use a PCA pump and a continuous infusion of morphine may be required. These patients are generally cared for in the ICU or HDU.

EPIDURAL INFUSIONS

Patients who had epidural anaesthesia may continue to receive analgesia by this route postoperatively. A low concentration of local anaesthetic (for example bupivacaine 0.125%) is combined with fentanyl (for example 4 µg/ml) and infused continuously into the epidural space. These patients must be cared for by staff used to dealing with such infusions. There is a risk of respiratory depression from the fentanyl and a rising dermatomal level of local anaesthetic block leading to hypotension and respiratory muscle weakness.

PRE-EMPTIVE ANALGESIA

It is assumed that preventing pain by blocking nociceptive stimulation as much as possible intraoperatively will reduce the severity of pain postoperatively, although proof of such an effect has been elusive. However, good intraoperative analgesia remains a part of balanced anaesthesia.

THE INTENSIVE CARE UNIT

The Intensive Care Unit (ICU) is the department that provides the highest level of continuous patient care and treatment. Recently, the concept of ICU has been replaced by that of Comprehensive Critical Care which includes ICU care, High Dependency Unit (HDU) care, and provision of specialist advice and support to other critically ill patients in the hospital by the Critical Care Outreach Team (CCOT).

The ICU provides:

- a nurse to patient ratio of 1:1
- a nurse in charge throughout 24 h
- 24-h cover by resident medical staff
- facilities to support organ system failures.

The HDU provides:
- a nurse to patient ratio of 1:2
- a nurse in charge throughout 24 h
- continuous availability of medical staff either from the admitting speciality or from ICU
- an appropriate level of monitoring and other equipment.

The CCOT aims to detect deterioration early and intervene to pre-empt the patient requiring admission to ICU/HDU. The aim is to prevent deterioration of patients on the wards to the point where severe morbidity or death is likely to occur, follow up ICU patients after discharge, and liaise between wards and ICU.

Patients should be referred immediately to the CCOT if they have:

- a compromised airway
- GCS ≤12
- FiO_2 >60% oxygen, or progressive increase in oxygen requirement
- arterial blood gas analysis showing:

  pH ≤7.2 or ≥7.55
  PaO_2 <8.0 kPa
  $PaCO_2$ >6.5 kPa.

Other potentially critically ill patients should be assessed regularly and those who deteriorate should be referred to CCOT.

GUIDELINES FOR ADMISSION AND DISCHARGE

ICU care must be directed towards those patients who are most likely to benefit:

- patients requiring, or likely to require, advanced respiratory support
- patients requiring support of two or more organ systems
- patients with co-morbidity who require support for an acute reversible failure of another organ system.

The types of organ support available are listed in Table 17.1.

The decision to admit or transfer a patient to an ICU or to refuse admission should be taken by senior medical staff. If the illness is non-reversible and incompatible with life then the patient should not be admitted. Occasionally it is necessary to admit patients and treat them appropriately for a period of time and assess any response. Subjecting a patient who is dying to ventilation and resuscitation merely to preserve organs for donation is neither ethical, moral nor legal.

TABLE 17.1 Categories of organ system support
1. Basic respiratory monitoring and support
More than 40% oxygen
Physiotherapy to clear secretions 2-hourly or more frequently
Recently extubated patients (after a prolonged period of intubation and ventilation)
Mask CPAP, or non-invasive ventilation
Patients who are intubated to protect their airway but do not need ventilation
2. Advanced respiratory support
Mechanical ventilatory support
Possibility of sudden deterioration in respiratory function requiring immediate intubation and mechanical ventilation
3. Circulatory support
Need for vasoactive drugs
Support for circulatory instability due to hypovolaemia unresponsive to modest volume replacement
After resuscitation from cardiac arrest when ICU or HDU care is considered appropriate
4. Neurological monitoring or support
CNS depression obtunding the airway and other protective reflexes
Invasive neurological monitoring
5. Renal support
Acute renal therapy

GUIDELINES FOR DISCHARGE

Patients should be discharged when the condition(s) that necessitated their admission have been successfully treated. They should be discharged to an appropriate level of care – either the HDU or the ward as determined by their clinical condition.

Approximately 25% of all patients will die on the ICU, often as a result of treatment limitation in the face of continued deterioration despite maximal appropriate supportive therapy. Palliative and compassionate care should be continued on the ICU if their death is imminent but where death is inevitable but likely to be delayed, they should be transferred to a non-ICU/HDU area for terminal care.

THE ROLE OF THE ICU RESIDENT

ASSESSMENT OF PATIENTS

When dealing with a newly admitted emergency patient assessment and resuscitation will often have to take place simultaneously and generally follows the standard pattern of recognizing and dealing with problems in the order of **A**irway, **B**reathing and **C**irculation.

THERAPEUTIC ACTION

The resident is the first doctor consulted by the nursing staff and must decide rapidly whether the problem is one they can deal with or if more experienced help is needed. The number of times when emergency action is needed should be relatively small when patients are continuously monitored by experienced ICU nurses, e.g. unforeseen circulatory collapse, accidental tracheal extubation.

COMMUNICATION

Patients may be under the care of several clinical teams and the ICU resident should act as the final common pathway for all changes in therapy. When the patient, relatives or friends are spoken to it is vital that the nurse is present and takes part in such discussions. The content of the discussion must be accurately recorded in the patient's notes.

CARDIAC ARREST AND TRAUMA TEAMS

In many hospitals the ICU resident is expected to attend all cardiac arrests and be a member of the Trauma Team in the Emergency Department. Ideally all ICU residents should be trained in Advanced Life Support (ALS) and Advanced Trauma Life Support (ATLS).

During in-hospital cardiac arrests the team is responsible for provision of advanced airway intervention and the diagnosis of the rhythm into either ventricular fibrillation/tachycardia (VF/VT) or non- VF/VT. The treatment then follows the Universal ALS Algorithm (see Figure 19.1, Action Plan 2).

Trauma resuscitation follows the principle of performing a Primary Survey (Table 17.2) – aiming to detect any immediately life threatening problems and carrying out simultaneous resuscitation. At the end of the Primary Survey, the following should have been achieved/performed:

- a secure airway
- protected cervical spine (if appropriate)
- oxygenation and ventilation
- insertion of two large bore intravenous lines
- control of compressible haemorrhage
- determination of the Glasgow Coma Score
- a complete external examination
- placement of adjuncts to diagnosis such as ECG, pulse oximeter and capnometry etc.

TABLE 17.2 Primary Survey

A – Airway and cervical spine control
B – Breathing, oxygenation and ventilation
C – Circulation and haemorrhage control
D – Disability
E – Exposure and environment

Following the Primary Survey and resuscitation a thorough Secondary Survey of the whole patient should be undertaken.

CLINICAL ASSESSMENT AND INITIAL MANAGEMENT

A thorough multi-system assessment is the key to appropriate management of patients admitted to the ICU. Often assessment and initial management run in parallel. Full patient assessment and examination of each patient, even if stable, should be carried out at least daily.

'ABC' BASED ASSESSMENT

A. Airway

- Is the airway patent and secure?
- Is the cervical spine at risk?
- Size, length and position of the tracheal tube?
- Is it time for a tracheostomy?
- What is coming up the tube?
- What is the cuff pressure?

B. Breathing

- Spontaneous ventilation: rate, depth, character
- Mechanical ventilation: what is the mode and what are the settings?
- Inspired oxygen concentration
- PEEP or CPAP level
- Position of the patient
- Clinical examination findings
- Are chest drains patent and swinging?
- Arterial blood gas analysis results
- Chest X-ray result.

C. Circulation

- ECG, pulse, blood pressure, CVP, pulmonary artery occlusion pressure
- Derived haemodynamic data, e.g. cardiac index
- Inotropes or other vasoactive agents
- Heart sounds
- Fluid balance, plasma osmolarity
- Peripheral circulation/oedema.

D. Disability/depth of sedation

- Sedation score or Glasgow Coma Score
- Dose of sedative agents
- Focal neurology, pupils (size, reactivity), fitting
- Cerebral function monitor results
- Other specialized neurological monitors, e.g. ICP, jugular bulb saturation or transcranial Doppler
- Imaging results.

E. Equipment

- Is it all working, calibrated and accurate?
- Is it in the right place, e.g. NG tubes in the stomach, CVP line tip not in the atrium?

F. Fluids

- Fluid balance over the previous 24 h, and cumulative
- Fluid output. Fistulae, drains, wounds 'output'
- What fluid to give.

G. Gut

- Stress ulcer prophylaxis
- Nasogastric tube aspirate/drainage
- Wounds healing or not?
- Stomas – viable, working or not?
- Bowel sounds present or bowels working?
- Abdominal distension from gas, fluid or blood. Is there any evidence of abdominal compartment syndrome?

H. Haematology

- Haematology, clotting, biochemistry and serology results
- Is transfusion required?

I. Imaging

- Are reports available?
- Is any further imaging required (including repeating existing imaging)?

J. Joints and limbs

- Fractures, dislocations, other trauma
- DVT prophylaxis – mechanical or low molecular weight heparin. Is DVT prophylaxis contraindicated?
- Peripheral pulses, perfusion and evidence of compartment syndrome.

K. Kelvin

- Temperature.

L. Lines

- When and where placed?
- Are they still required?
- Signs of sepsis. Blood cultures from lines.

M. Microbiology

- Aggressive microbiological surveillance: swabs, blood cultures, sputum, bronchi-alveolar lavage or undirected catheter lavage (better than simple sputum sampling), drain fluid, urine, removed line tips
- Strict asepsis and cross infection avoidance – 'Touch a patient – wash your hands'. Always wear gloves and an apron when examining patients
- If possible isolate patients with resistant organisms
- Directed antimicrobial therapy only
- Antibiotic levels, doses and course duration.

N. Nutrition

- Type of feeding
- Dietary supplements
- Check trace elements
- Blood sugar control.

O. Other Consultants

- Are further opinions needed?
- Inform the General Practitioner that the patient has been admitted.

P. Pain relief, psychological support, prescriptions

- Its analgesia adequate?
- Talk to patient even if they have a depressed level of consciousness.
- Explain procedures simply and carefully.
- Sedation and psychotropic drugs, if indicated.
- Review drug charts.

Q. Questions

- If you are unsure of what to do, ask your Consultant.
- Never undertake a task in which you have been inadequately trained.

R. Relatives

- Keep relatives fully informed.
- Always hold discussions away from the bedside unless the patient is fully aware or autonomous and can participate.
- Always hold discussions in the presence of the patient's nurse and document your comments.

S. Skin
- Examine skin for perfusion, wounds, and signs of systemic disease or infection.
- Pressure area care, mouth care etc.

T. Trauma and Transport
- Is the Secondary Survey complete?
- Transport of ICU patients within or between hospitals requires the same level of care and monitoring that they receive on the ICU itself.

U. Universal precautions
- Wear gloves and aprons.
- Use additional precautions when performing invasive procedures.

V. Visitors
- Treat patient's relatives or other medical personnel with respect and courtesy.

W. What to do
- Once the patient has been fully assessed you must formulate a plan to deal with the patient's problems.
- This plan must be documented clearly in the notes and discussed with the bedside nurse.
- Parameters must be agreed within which the nurse is able to vary the components of the therapeutic regime according to the patient's response and outside which you need to re-assess the patient.
- Time is an important part of your plan and regular re-assessment is essential.

Y. Why?
- Every time you review the patient ask yourself why the patient was admitted and what are their active problems now.
- Keep on track and forget nothing!

CARE BUNDLES

A recent change in the provision of care is the use of 'Care Bundles' where several evidence-based techniques are used in combination in the hope that they will be synergistic and result in reduced mortality. The most widely used care bundle relates to ventilatory support. This combines a lung protective ventilatory strategy, low tidal volumes, PEEP and recruitment, permissive hypercarbia, semi-recumbent patient positioning, intermittent sedation 'holidays' and protocol driven weaning. A Care Bundle for sepsis has been developed by the Surviving Sepsis Campaign. This includes the ventilation bundle combined with strict glycaemic control, steroid therapy, early diagnosis, measurement of lactate levels, early antibiotic therapy with fluid resuscitation +/– inotropic support aimed at achieving a central venous oxygen saturation of greater than 70%.

GENERAL CARE OF CRITICALLY ILL PATIENTS

Apart from specific organ (system) monitoring and support certain general elements of care, common to all patients, are provided:

- Skin care
- Airway clearance (tracheal suction)
- Stress ulcer prophylaxis
- DVT prophylaxis
- Turning patients to prevent development of pressure areas
- Washing, eye, mouth and bowel care
- Mobilization and passive movement
- Sedation and analgesia
- Attention to nutrition
- Prevention of cross infection
- Psychological support to patients and relatives.

All these measures take considerable patience and skill and are important contributors to good outcome.

Most patients require some sedation and/or analgesia. Ideally, patients should receive only light sedation, except when unpleasant or painful procedures are performed, so that they can understand and cooperate with therapy. Regular assessment and formal sedation scoring such as the Ramsay Sedation Scale (Table 17.3) should be performed. A range of sedatives are available and should be combined with analgesics and given by continuous infusion. Examples include morphine and midazolam, and propofol and alfentanil. Very few patients require neuromuscular blockade in addition to sedation and analgesia.

All ICU patients need feeding and most are unable to take a normal diet. Early enteral nutrition improves outcome and there is some evidence that certain dietary supplements such as glutamine

TABLE 17.3 Ramsay Sedation Scale for sedation

Score	Clinical signs
1	Patient is anxious and agitated or restless, or both
2	Patient is cooperative, oriented, and tranquil
3	Patient responds to commands only
4	Patient exhibits brisk response to light glabellar tap or loud auditory stimulus
5	Patient exhibits a sluggish response to light glabellar tap or loud auditory stimulus
6	Patient exhibits no response

may improve immune function and survival. Parenteral feeding will be required in patients unsuitable for enteral feeding:

- gastro-intestinal obstruction
- prolonged paralytic ileus
- short bowel syndrome
- entero-cutaneous fistulae

 Sepsis is involved in the majority of late deaths (>5 days).

Cross infection is a particular risk and strict asepsis and personal hygiene is vital. The emergence of multi-resistant micro-organisms is an increasing problem and is best conquered by control of cross infection, good aseptic techniques and microbiological surveillance on a regular basis with swabs, blood cultures and other samples being taken at every opportunity. The widespread use of prophylactic or broad-spectrum antibiotics is avoided.

TRANSFERS

Anaesthetists are often involved in transporting ICU patients to other areas within the hospital or to other hospitals. This should not be undertaken without adequate preparation and training. The decision to transfer to another hospital is the joint responsibility of the referring doctor, receiving doctor and the transfer personnel. If the patient requires intensive care then the authority to accept the patient must rest with the ICU Consultant at the receiving hospital. The mode of transfer depends on the reason for transfer, the urgency of transfer, the distance of transfer, the time taken to arrange personnel and vehicle, weather and traffic conditions. All escorts must be appropriately trained and should pay meticulous attention to resuscitation and stabilization. Objective evidence of adequate oxygenation and ventilation (PaO_2 >13 kPa, $PaCO_2$ 4.0–4.5 kPa, SaO_2 >95%), and objective evidence of cardiovascular stability (systolic BP >120 mmHg, pulse <120/min, urine output >40 ml/h), must be achieved before starting the transfer.

> ⚠ **The patient must be fully resuscitated and stabilized prior to transfer. Never undertake a transfer of a patient who is persistently shocked despite attempts at resuscitation.**

The rules for safe transfer are listed in Table 17.4.

The following head-injured patients require tracheal intubation prior to transfer:

● GCS ≤8, or deteriorating GCS on repeated assessment
● Depressed laryngeal reflexes
● PaO_2 < 9 kPa on air or < 13 kPa on oxygen
● $PaCO_2$ > 6 kPa or abnormal respiratory pattern
● Potential for airway compromise from bleeding from the nose or mouth, mandibular fractures
● Seizure activity.

A nasogastric tube and urinary catheter should be inserted and left on free drainage. Wounds and burns must be dressed with non-constrictive dressings and unstable fractures stabilized. In trauma patients the cervical spine must remain fully immobilized until its

---

TABLE 17.4 Rules for safe transfers

If in doubt intubate and ventilate the patient's lungs prior to transfer (rather than attempting to do it in transit).
Drain pneumothoraces prior to transfer.
Chest drains should be of the flutter-valve type rather than underwater seals and must not be clamped at any time during transfer.
Secure all tubes entering the patient – for example tracheal, chest drainage, venous or arterial lines.
Ensure adequate sedation and analgesia.
Every time you move the patient check the tubes and lines

TABLE 17.5 Equipment for transfer of critically ill patients

Portable ventilator with high and low pressure alarms, disconnection alarm, variable FiO_2, provision of PEEP, CPAP and various ventilatory modes.

Adequate supplies of pressurized oxygen. *Make sure you have the correct spanner to turn on replacement cylinders!*

Self-inflating bag and Ambu-valve as a back-up.

Monitor for ECG, non-invasive and intra-arterial blood pressure

Capnography in ventilated patients

Temperature monitor

Portable defibrillator

Suction unit

---

integrity has been confirmed using ATLS guidelines. The patient's notes, blood results, blood or blood products for use in transit, X-rays and any other documentation must accompany the patient. The standard of monitoring should be identical to that during routine Intensive Care. The monitors themselves must accompany the patient at all stages of their journey. A list of recommended equipment is given in Table 17.5.

The full range of resuscitation drugs, sedatives, analgesics, muscle relaxants and appropriate intravenous anaesthetic agents are required together with the necessary syringe pumps, power sources, cannulae, syringes, fluids etc. The Transfer Team must dress appropriately for the environment. A portable phone, together with referring and receiving hospital phone numbers for use in emergencies is essential, although the risk of electrical interference must be considered prior to its use. A pre-transfer checklist is given in Table 17.6.

TABLE 17.6 Pre-transfer checklist

Equipment, batteries, oxygen, fluids and drugs checked and ready?

Transfer vehicle ready and waiting?

Reception at receiving hospital confirmed with named doctor, estimated time of arrival given to receiving hospital?

Confirmed bed still available and its exact location?

All case notes, results, referral letter collected?

Contact numbers and phone?

Return arrangements checked?

Relatives informed of departure?

Is the patient still stable after transfer to trolley?

Equipment, tubes and lines still attached and functioning?

PRACTICAL CLINICAL GUIDELINES FOR ORGAN SUPPORT

RESPIRATORY SUPPORT

Any patient who develops hypoxaemia and/or hypercapnia may be a candidate for respiratory support provided that their pulmonary pathology is potentially reversible. There is a range or respiratory support from simple mask oxygen therapy to sophisticated mechanical modes of ventilation (Table 17.7). The correct treatment depends upon the patient's clinical condition and on the potential for deterioration. For example – arterial blood gases may be normal but the patient may be on the point of exhaustion.

Hypoxaemia

Hypoxaemia occurs when areas of the lung have greater pulmonary blood flow than alveolar ventilation and blood flow is said to be 'shunted'. Hypoxaemia caused by this mechanism shows little improvement when the inspired oxygen concentration is increased. If moderate anaemia (Hb <10 g/dl) is present, as it is in many ICU patients, severe hypoxaemia (PaO_2 <6 kPa) may occur without obvious cyanosis.

Oxygen therapy and continuous positive airway pressure (CPAP)

All critically ill patients need humidified oxygen in appropriate concentrations. Low-concentration fixed-performance masks delivering 24–35% oxygen should be reserved for use by those patients with chronic lung conditions in whom hypoxia is maintaining respiratory drive. Such patients are very rare in ICU practice.

TABLE 17.7 Range of modalities for respiratory support

Oxygen therapy with face-mask
Oxygen therapy with face-mask using high gas flow
Continuous positive airway pressure (CPAP) mask
Non-invasive supplementation of respiration
Tracheal intubation and intermittent positive pressure ventilation (IPPV)
IPPV with positive end-expiratory pressure (PEEP)
Different modes of ventilation allowing patient participation – Assisted Spontaneous Breathing (ASB), Pressure Support Ventilation (PSV)
Pressure-controlled modes with variable I : E ratios
High frequency ventilation/oscillation

Oxygen therapy should be continuously monitored by pulse oximetry and by blood gas analysis after 30 min and regularly thereafter. If patients remain hypoxaemic despite oxygen delivery by face-mask, or if they are breathless (in particular with a diagnosis of chronic obstructive airway disease or pulmonary oedema), then Continuous Positive Airway Pressure (CPAP) by mask should be tried if there are no contraindications (Table 17.8). A tightly applied face-mask with a high volume, low pressure, soft plastic rim held in place by a special harness is connected to a circuit delivering an air/oxygen mixture of the required FiO_2. The flow of fresh gas in the circuit must be sufficient to keep the positive pressure set by the expiratory valve (2.5–10 cmH$_2$O) almost constant throughout the respiratory cycle with only minimal negative pressure drop during inspiration. For CPAP to be successful, the patient must have adequate analgesia, be alert and cooperative. The benefits of CPAP are:

- improved functional residual capacity – reduction in shunt and better oxygenation
- improved respiratory mechanics – less exhaustion
- some reduction in the total lung water.

The advantages of CPAP are:

- patients remain spontaneously breathing
- it is non-invasive
- minimal sedation required
- patients can actively participate in physiotherapy.

The disadvantages are:

- not suitable for unconscious patients
- not suitable for patients at risk of aspiration
- gastric distension (requirement for nasogastric tube)
- noisy
- the face-mask may be uncomfortable and cause pressure sores. (Consider nasal CPAP).

TABLE 17.8 Contraindications to CPAP

Facial injuries
Basal skull fractures
Unconscious patient
Uncooperative patient
Severe respiratory failure

Hypercapnia

Carbon dioxide clearance is determined by alveolar ventilation and any disease that decreases minute ventilation may cause 'type 2' respiratory failure. In end-stage lung disease intubation and ventilation is not appropriate. For some patients non-invasive (i.e. non-intubational) forms of respiratory support are applicable: for example non-invasive positive pressure ventilation by mask (NIPPV). Failure of non-invasive support is suggested if the $PaCO_2$ continues to rise or exceeds 8 kPa after 2 h of treatment. A rapid respiratory rate with shallow breathing is often the first sign of impending exhaustion and deterioration in the level of consciousness occurs rapidly once the $PaCO_2$ starts to rise above 8 kPa.

Institution of mechanical ventilation

The indications for mechanical ventilation are:
- PaO_2 <8 kPa despite oxygen therapy
- unsuccessful application of CPAP or non-invasive ventilation
- decreased level of consciousness
- airway compromise requiring tracheal intubation.

Tracheal intubation

If the patient is conscious, anaesthesia should be induced carefully with an appropriate dose of an intravenous induction agent and muscle relaxant using a rapid sequence technique with pre-oxygenation and cricoid pressure. Critically ill patients are often exquisitely sensitive to intravenous induction agents. Intubation in head injured patients requires a technique that prevents an increase in intracranial pressure during laryngoscopy and intubation. If the patient is unconscious and the victim of blunt trauma, cervical spine injury is a possibility and the cervical spine should be immobilized during intubation using manual in-line immobilization (MILI).

Naso-tracheal intubation is usually avoided in the ICU because of the increased incidence of sepsis from sinusitis. A chest X-ray should be taken to ensure that the tip of the tube lies at least 5 cm above the carina. Endobronchial intubation is a common complication during prolonged mechanical ventilation as the tracheal tube may migrate down the trachea when the patient is moved for normal nursing procedures.

The complications of tracheal intubation and mechanical ventilation are listed in Table 17.9. Cardiac output may be reduced by the decrease in preload caused by positive intra-thoracic pressure

---

TABLE 17.9 Complications of tracheal intubation and mechanical ventilation

Barotrauma – pneumothorax, pneumomediastinum
Endobronchial intubation
Atelectasis, sputum retention and infection
Ventilation/perfusion mismatch
Reduced venous return and hypotension
Decreased glomerular filtration and oliguria
Increased secretion of antidiuretic hormone
Sodium retention
Reduction in splanchnic blood flow

---

during IPPV. This effect is particularly marked if the patient is hypo-volaemic, elderly, or has myocardial dysfunction.

Modes of ventilation

The basic mode of ventilation – controlled mandatory ventilation (CMV) – is used during balanced anaesthesia, but it is rarely used on the ICU. Most ICUs use a mode of ventilation that allows the patient to take breaths if they are able to do so. Suppression of the patient's spontaneous respiratory efforts by prolonged deep sedation with or without neuromuscular blockade may result in atrophy of the respiratory muscles leading to prolonged weaning. In synchronized intermittent mandatory ventilation (SIMV) the patient's own respiratory efforts are detected and synchronized with machine breaths. The patient's own respiratory efforts are supported in pressure support ventilation (PSV). PSV is essentially patient triggered, pressure-limited ventilation and can only be used if the patient has a normal intrinsic respiratory rate. These techniques allow:

- less sedation
- preservation of respiratory muscle tone
- greater cardiovascular stability
- prevention of the surges in airway pressure which would occur if a mandatory inspiratory breath was imposed by the ventilator when the patient was trying to breathe out.

The common problems encountered in ventilated patients, irrespective of the mode of ventilation, are given in Table 17.10.

A summary of a strategy for respiratory support is given in Table 17.11. Patients should be ventilated for the shortest possible period of time because of the detrimental effects of prolonged intubation, ventilation and sedation. The process of gradually decreasing the amount of ventilatory support to reach unsupported spontaneous breathing is known as weaning.

TABLE 17.10 Common problems during mechanical ventilation

Low airway pressure

Disconnection or leak in circuit
Sudden increase in lung compliance

High airway pressure

Blocked or misplaced tube
Endobronchial intubation
Bronchospasm
Asynchronous breathing
Pneumothorax
Splinting of the diaphragm by abdominal compartment pressure

Low tidal volume

Disconnection or leak
Asynchronous breathing
Bronchospasm
Sputum retention
Splinting of diaphragm
Pneumothorax
Any other cause of decreased lung compliance

Sudden hypoxaemia

FiO_2 too low
Circuit leak
Tube misplacement to oesophagus or right main bronchus
Pneuomothorax
Severe bronchospasm
Progressive pulmonary pathology

Sudden hypercarbia

Worsening pulmonary pathology
Decreased tidal volume or respiratory rate or loss of minute ventilation by circuit leak
Overproduction of CO_2, e.g. during high fever, asynchronous breathing

Action

To find out if it is a ventilator or patient problem, 'bag' the patient with 100% O_2, *look* for chest movement, *listen* for breath sounds and *feel* for changes in lung compliance.

CARDIOVASCULAR SUPPORT

Disorders of the cardiovascular system (CVS) are very common in ICU patients and may be due to primary cardiac disease, co-morbidity from other medical conditions, e.g. sepsis, diabetes or renal failure, or from complications following surgical procedures. Any disorder causing reduced efficiency of the cardiovascular system may result in inadequate delivery of oxygen to the tissues

---

TABLE 17.11 Summary of a strategy to provide respiratory support

1. Consider trial of CPAP
2. Look for signs of failure to respond:
   - increased respiratory rate
   - dyspnoea
   - inability to talk in complete sentences
   - hypercapnia and/or hypoxaemia
3. Consider the use of non-invasive ventilatory techniques
4. Intubate and ventilate. Use assisted spontaneous modes wherever possible
5. If failure of oxygenation occurs and FiO_2 >0.6, convert to a pressure-controlled, inverse ratio mode with PEEP
6. Accept low tidal volumes and permissive hypercapnia
7. Use the prone position if oxygenation fails to improve. Avoid oxygen toxicity and set realistic goals for oxygenation, e.g. SaO_2 >90%
8. Consider inhaled nitric oxide or prostacycline
9. Prevent atelectasis by regular turning and physiotherapy
10. Meticulous fluid balance to minimize extravascular lung water
11. Effective sedation at lowest possible doses

---

for their metabolic needs, initiating a cascade of events that leads to organ failure. The causes of cardiovascular disturbance include too little volume, too much volume, primary 'pump' problems, afterload too high and afterload too low.

Disordered cardiovascular function may be well compensated at first leading to apparently 'normal' or only slightly deranged pulse rate and blood pressure. Assessment of the cardiovascular system (Table 17.12) must be systematic, accurately documented and repeated following any intervention, e.g. fluid administration.

TABLE 17.12 Cardiovascular assessment in critical care

Examination of general condition
Respiratory rate, FiO_2 oxygen saturation, arterial blood gases
Heart rate and rhythm
Systemic blood pressure – systolic and diastolic
Chest X-ray
CVP
Advanced CVS monitoring, e.g. cardiac output
Temperature
Urinary output
Lines – position and condition
Fluid therapy
Drainage from fistulae, wounds etc.
Review of drug chart for drugs known to have CVS effects

Additional investigations such as full blood count, clotting screen and urea and electrolytes should be regarded as routine in all ICU patients and additional focused investigations such as troponin I levels are used when myocardial injury is suspected. The chest X-ray may demonstrate features directly related to cardiac disease or conditions associated with disordered cardiac function:

- air in pleural cavity
- air or blood in pericardium
- bleeding into chest cavity
- pulmonary oedema or other abnormalities of lung tissue
- collections of fluid in the pleural cavity or lung tissue.

A 12-lead ECG should be performed in all patients newly admitted to ICU. This will act as a baseline for comparison with any subsequent cardiac events that may occur and may also demonstrate co-existing cardiac disease. One of the commonest cardiac problems in ICU patients is the sudden emergence of an irregular heart rhythm which may be related to causes other than primary cardiac disease (Table 17.13).

Diagnosis of different types of shock

Hypovolaemic, septic, cardiogenic, anaphylactic and neurogenic shock are all seen in the ICU and require different treatments. To aid diagnosis you should ask:

- Is there an obvious cause such as visible haemorrhage or other fluid loss?
- Is there any deficit between fluid input and fluid output?
- Has the patient complained of chest pain or has a history of cardiac problems?
- Is there a high or low temperature, high or low white blood cell count, history of recent surgery or other cause of sepsis?

TABLE 17.13 Non-cardiac causes of dysrrhythmia

Hypoxia
Hypercapnia
Hyper- or hypokalaemia
Hypomagnesaemia
Hypovolaemia
Metabolic acidosis
Pro-arryhtmogenic drugs
Irritation of myocardium by tip of CPV line in right atrium or pulmonary artery catheter
Cardiac or pulmonary surgery

- Is there a spinal cord injury?
- Has the patient collapsed during drug administration?

The initial treatment of most forms of shock will involve the provision of oxygen and fluid therapy. There is no convincing evidence
that either colloid or crystalloid fluid replacement has a specific
advantage over the other. The physiological endpoints of volume
resuscitation are also unclear. The aim should be to balance both
preload and afterload to give the optimum cardiac output.

Simple clinical methods of monitoring the CVS such as pulse
rate, capillary refill, blood pressure or surrogate markers of cardiac
output such as urine output are not sufficiently sensitive to record
the rapid changes that occur in seriously ill patients. Invasive
monitoring such as arterial lines, central venous lines and, occasionally, a pulmonary artery flotation catheter (PAC) may be used.
Intra-arterial catheters provide a more accurate and 'beat to beat'
measurement of blood pressure.

Central venous pressure monitoring

Multi-lumen central lines provide separate access for the drug infusions and allow measurement of central venous pressure (CVP). The
CVP is often used as a surrogate marker of intravascular volume
but has limitations. In hypovolaemia it may be low, normal or high
depending on the degree of compensatory vasoconstriction caused
by catecholamines or hypothermia. A high CVP could be due to
high pulmonary artery pressure, pulmonary pathology or high intra-
thoracic pressure rather than as a result of cardiac failure or volume
overload. Trends over time and changes in response to fluid chal-
lenges are more reliable than single readings. Indications for intensive
CVS monitoring are summarized in Table 17.14.

Pulmonary artery catheters

Use of PACs is decreasing in ICU and is being replaced by non-
invasive methods of estimation of cardiac output such as transoesophageal Doppler (TOE). PAC catheters provide information
on:

- cardiac output
- pulmonary artery pressure
- pulmonary artery occlusion (or 'wedge') pressure
- systemic and pulmonary vascular resistance
- mixed venous oxygen saturation
- oxygen consumption
- delivery and extraction of oxygen.

> **TABLE 17.14 Indications for intensive CVS monitoring**
> - To balance afterload and preload, e.g. severe sepsis or cardiogenic shock
> - Rapid fluid shifts, e.g. major haemorrhage, severe pancreatitis, large surface area burns
> - Use of vasoactive drugs such as inotropes or vasodilators to manipulate afterload and myocardial contractility

Complications of insertion and use of a PAC are described in Table 17.15. The measurement of pulmonary artery occlusion pressure is taken as a surrogate marker of left ventricular end-diastolic volume. For this to be true there must be normal left ventricular compliance, normal end-diastolic pressure, normal mitral valve function, normal left atrial pressure and normal intra-thoracic pressure and pulmonary vasculature. In general, if correctly placed in the absence of high PEEP, a pulmonary artery occlusion pressure more than 18 mmHg indicates volume overload while a pressure less than 12 mmHg indicates relative hypovolaemia.

Trans-oesophageal echocardiography/Doppler

A Doppler ultrasound probe is placed in the oesophagus to lie alongside the descending aorta and allows the continuous measurement of velocity waveforms. The area under the recorded waveform can be equated to stroke volume using a nomogram. Information

> **TABLE 17.15 Complications of pulmonary artery flotation catheter use**
>
> Infection
> Thrombosis
> Pneumothorax
> Arterial puncture
> Haemothorax
> Neuropraxia
> Air embolism
> Dysrrhythmias
> Catheter embolism
> Pulmonary infarction
> Pulmonary artery rupture
> Knotting of the catheter within the heart
> Sterile endocarditis
> Cardiac perforation

on cardiac output, circulating volume and peripheral resistance can also be derived.

Pulse contour analysis

The peripheral arterial pulse waveform is a function of the cardiac output, the peripheral vascular resistance, peripheral vascular compliance and the arterial pressure. If the cardiac output is measured for a given peripheral arterial waveform, then after calibration, changes in the peripheral pulse waveform can be used to calculate changes in the cardiac output. The LiDCO and PiCCO systems use intermittent cardiac output determination using a specific indicator to calibrate the continuous pulse waveform analysis.

RENAL SUPPORT

Renal failure and oliguria are very common in ICU patients – often as a part of multiple organ failure. Prevention of dysfunction progressing to established renal failure depends upon preservation of adequate perfusion and oxygenation. A strategy to manage renal dysfunction is given in Table 17.16.

The indications for renal replacement therapy are given in Table 17.17 and the management of hyperkalaemia is described in Table 17.18.

TABLE 17.16 Strategy to manage renal dysfunction

- Ensure an adequate cardiac output, perfusion pressure and intravascular volume
- Only use diuretics after intravascular volume and cardiac output have been optimized
- Sudden cessation of urinary output should be regarded as due to obstruction until proved otherwise
- Review all drugs regularly for possible nephrotoxic effects
- Modify doses of drugs relying on renal elimination
- Treat hyperkalaemia by acute potassium lowering methods until definitive renal support can be arranged (see Table 17.18)
- In patients with rhabdomyolysis use aggressive fluid loading combined with alkalinization and mannitol
- Loop diuretic infusions in non-oliguric renal failure may reduce distal tubular oxygen consumption, and preserve high volume, but poor quality urine output

---

TABLE 17.17 Indications for renal replacement therapy

- Uncontrollable hyperkalaemia (K^+ >6 mmol/l) or academia (BE > −10 mmol/l)
- Severe oliguria or anuria when compulsory therapeutic fluid requirement (e.g. blood or blood products, parenteral nutrition and drug volume) input exceeds output
- High urea (>35–40 mmol/l) or creatinine (>350–400 μmol/l)
- To correct very high sodium levels in a controlled manner
- To correct severe volume overload

TABLE 17.18 Emergency management of hyperkalaemia

- Calcium chloride 10%, 10 ml, slowly i.v. (5 min)
- Glucose 50%, 50 ml plus soluble insulin 10 i.u., over 15–30 min
- Sodium bicarbonate 8.4%, 50 ml slow i.v. (5–10 min)
- Haemofiltration or dialysis

NEUROSURGICAL INTENSIVE CARE

The aim of intensive care in neurosurgical patients is to prevent secondary injury caused by hypoxia, hypotension, hypercarbia and metabolic disturbance. The goals are to keep the environment of the brain as normal as possible (Table 17.19).

Cerebral perfusion pressure (CPP) calculation requires direct measurement of intracranial pressure (ICP) and MAP:

$$CPP = MAP - ICP$$

The ICP should be maintained at normal levels (<10 mmHg) and untoward swings in response to stimulation prevented by adequate sedation and analgesia. CPP may be elevated with judicious fluid loading to normovolaemia and the use of pressor

---

TABLE 17.19 Goals of neurological critical care

- Maintain normoxia and normocapnia (PaO_2 >12 kPa and $PaCO_2$ 4–5 kPa)
- Avoid prolonged hyperventilation ($PaCO_2$ <3.5 kPa)
- Normotension and preservation of CPP >60 mmHg
- Normoglycaemia
- Prevent hypernatraemia and maintain plasma osmolality <315 mosmol/l
- Intubation and sedation if airway protection required
- Cool to normothermia if pyrexial

agents, e.g. norepinephrine. This technique may be detrimental in those patients who have lost the power to autoregulate as it may provoke increased tissue fluid formation. Persistently raised ICP may respond to increasing doses of intravenous anaesthetic agents (but not ketamine), muscle relaxation or surface cooling to induce hypothermia (34.5°C) in an attempt to decrease cerebral metabolic rate.

Transcranial Doppler determination of cerebral blood flow velocity, jugular venous bulb oxygen saturation or oxygen electrodes placed within the brain substance itself may be used to provide information about cerebral blood flow and oxygenation. Brain electrical activity may be monitored by compressed spectral array or the cerebral function analysis monitor.

PREPARING FOR A CAREER IN ANAESTHESIA

At the outset of a career in anaesthesia, the new trainee needs to focus upon what will be required of him or her professionally, and how to make the most of the available training opportunities. These areas will be considered under the following headings:

- The organization of specialist training in the UK
- Obtaining a training post in anaesthesia in the UK
- The novice anaesthetist
- Understanding educational processes
- Professional development
- Understanding management issues
- The Primary FRCA (Fellowship of the Royal College of Anaesthetists) Examination
- The requirements for entry into Higher Specialist Training/ Specialist Registrar grade
- Further reading.

THE ORGANIZATION OF SPECIALIST TRAINING IN THE UK

It is increasingly recognized that meeting the educational needs of trainees during the early years of their professional careers is important, not least because high quality patient care depends on sound education and training from the outset. At the time of writing specialist training is undergoing significant modernization with recognition that although the apprenticeship model remains the basis for medical training, it needs to be efficiently managed and quality-assured and there is a key change of direction towards outcome-based learning. The changes in training are part of the *Modernizing Medical Careers* initiative put forward by the Health Departments of the four UK home countries – and the reader should access their website (www.mmc.nhs.uk) for the most up-to-date information.

In the first two years following graduation, doctors will enter a broad-based two year Foundation Programme. The educational aims for the Foundation Programme will be to develop generic skills, competencies and attitudes relevant to any future medical career. The Foundation Programme trainee will undertake a series of structured assessments. These are intended to confirm that the educational aims have been successfully met and the trainee is suitable to progress further in postgraduate medical training. After the Foundation Programme, doctors will be eligible to apply for a Specialist Training Programme of their choice. It is likely that experience and feedback from the Foundation Programme will inform the career choices of trainees in planning for their next stage of training. As the *Modernizing Medical Careers* initiative moves towards full implementation, it is anticipated that from August 2007 Specialist Training Programmes will become seamless with a single run-through training programme. The first two years of a Specialist Training programme (ST1 and ST2) will be equivalent to the basic specialist SHO training currently in place at the time of writing. As long as the trainees in years ST1 and ST2 make satisfactory progress and meet the examination requirements, they will continue into Higher Specialist Training without having to overcome further hurdles. It is also anticipated that another kind of specialist training post will also be available: the fixed term training post. These posts will also provide competency-based training in anaesthesia. The content and delivery of this training is likely to be very similar or identical to that of ST1 and ST2 trainees. However, trainees in these posts will only gain access to higher training by competing for any vacancies which may arise at year ST3.

TABLE 18.1 Training roles and responsibilities

Role	Responsibilities
Postgraduate Dean	Overall management of postgraduate training at a local level Formulation of educational contracts with hospitals Ensuring trainee well-being, helping the trainee with problems
Programme Director	Acts as the Postgraduate Dean's representative in the School of Anaesthesia Responsible for managing specialist training
College Tutor	The local point of contact with the Royal College of Anaesthetists Local organization of training with programme director Oversees examination preparation Facilitates professional development of the trainee
Educational Supervisor	Agrees learning needs with the trainee Monitors the progress towards achieving objectives Validates the learning achievement by confirming satisfactory progress
Regional Advisor	Monitors training throughout the region on behalf of the College

The generic content of early training, regardless of speciality, has been set out by the General Medical Council (GMC) in the document 'The Early Years' (see Further Reading) and the local Postgraduate Dean oversees this. The specialist content of training in anaesthesia has been set out by The Royal College of Anaesthetists (RCA) which, in conjunction with the Postgraduate Medical Education and Training Board (PMETB) is responsible for overseeing specialist training in anaesthesia. There are a number of key figures in the planning and delivery of the training programme (see Table 18.1).

OBTAINING A TRAINING POST IN ANAESTHESIA IN THE UK

Appointment to an initial training post in anaesthesia is the first hurdle to be cleared when planning a career in the speciality. Novice anaesthetists are virtually unique in medicine in that their first three months are devoted almost entirely to training rather than service. This places demands on the provision of service locally, and consequently the supply of these posts is limited and they are often highly sought after.

The intention of *Modernizing Medical Careers* is that entry into Specialist Training will be by a competitive process. At the time of writing it is unclear exactly what form this process will take. The intention is that it should be open, fair, flexible and competitive, and carried out according to clear, uniform UK-wide principles. The selection process will be key to successful Specialist Training as it will be necessary to select applicants with the personal and professional attributes required to work successfully as an anaesthetist. Pilot projects have explored the use of Assessment Centres for this task and it is unlikely that in the future a traditional panel interview will be used to select trainees.

For applicants from outside the UK the process for appointment to a UK training post within MMC is not fully formalized at the time of writing. Successful applicants will need to provide evidence that they have achieved competencies equivalent to those of the UK Foundation Programme. A successful application may depend on other factors such as other post-registration experience, academic achievement, postgraduate qualifications including Life Support Provider status, participation in and understanding of clinical audit, and good communication skills.

THE NOVICE ANAESTHETIST

Having secured a training post, the novice anaesthetist enters one of the most intensive training periods of his or her professional life. The trainee will receive one-to-one clinical teaching from consultant trainers and a high level of clinical supervision. During these early weeks, the new anaesthetists rapidly acquire new skills and knowledge. Much of this time is spent in the operating theatre, but emphasis is also placed on the role of the anaesthetist in perioperative care. Learning about preoperative assessment and postoperative management is given high priority from the beginning.

COLLEGE REGISTRATION

In the UK, the Certificate of Training (CCT) is awarded to doctors in training by the Postgraduate Medical Education and Training Board (PMETB). The CCT in anaesthesia is awarded on the recommendation of the RCA when the training programme has been successfully completed. If a post is recognized by the RCA for training, it will have been assessed to ensure appropriate quality and content of training. If a trainee wishes to claim their training in anaesthesia towards the award of a CCT, he or she *must* register with the RCA. RCA registration forms can be obtained from the local College Tutor or downloaded from the College website.

After registration with the RCA the trainee will be sent:

- A unique RCA reference number.
- The RCA manual for SHO Training: 'The CCST in Anaesthesia II: Competency Based Senior House Officer Training and Assessment'.
- Information about logbooks and examination regulations.
- Information about RCA educational activities.
- The College Bulletin.
- The British Journal of Anaesthesia.

LOGBOOK

All anaesthetic trainees are required to keep a logbook of cases. Examination of logbooks is an important part of formal assessment. The details of all anaesthetic activity should be recorded and many trainees use an electronic form of data collection from which summaries may be generated. The RCA website contains information about logbooks and also software programmes which may be downloaded and used for data collection and analysis.

THE SHO TRAINING MANUAL – 'THE CCST II: COMPETENCY BASED SENIOR HOUSE OFFICER TRAINING AND ASSESSMENT'

This training guide published by the RCA describes the programme of training for SHOs in the UK. It sets out the competencies that should be achieved in the first two years of training. It also describes the methods for assessing that the trainee has achieved these competencies, and it contains the syllabus for the Primary FRCA Examination.

UNDERSTANDING EDUCATIONAL PROCESSES

SERVICE-BASED LEARNING

Doctors in training grades must balance their educational needs with the service commitment to their department and patients. Much training depends on experiential or practice-based learning.

- In order to make the most of clinical experience, every service commitment should be regarded as a potential learning opportunity.
- The trainee should learn to think systematically about each clinical experience and develop reflective practice.
- The trainee should develop skills of self-evaluation; this is aided by seeking informal feedback from trainers.

Service-based learning may, by its nature, be haphazard and difficult to plan. Some hospitals aim to enhance systematic service-based learning by using training modules.

SUPERVISION

Appropriate clinical and educational supervision is a key principle of training.

Clinical supervision
To protect the interests of patients and trainees, systems should be in place to ensure that at all times the trainee has direct access to

a more senior colleague for assistance and advice. Trainees should never be burdened with clinical responsibilities too great for their level of experience or expertise.

The RCA recognizes three different levels of supervision:

- Immediately available: the supervisor is actually with the trainee or can be, within seconds of being called.
- Local: the supervisor is on the same geographical site, is immediately available for advice and is able to be with the trainee within 10 minutes of being called.
- Distant: the supervisor is rapidly available for advice but is separated from the trainee by more than 10 minutes.

Clinical supervision may be provided by a Consultant or a more senior trainee.

Educational supervision

The educational supervisor will:

- Agree clinical and non-clinical learning needs with the trainee.
- Agree a plan to achieve the learning objectives.
- Monitor the performance of the trainee and their progress towards achieving their objectives.
- Validate the learning achievement, usually by use of a standardized report form.

Educational supervisors are responsible for identifying substandard performance and work with the College Tutor and Postgraduate Dean to put remedial measures in place.

ASSESSMENT

Supervisors have a responsibility to ensure that doctors in training are competent to perform the tasks expected of them and patient safety must never be compromised by so-called learning curves. As training is competency-based, there is a requirement both for an assessment of competence and a documentation of this process. Clinical competence depends on:

- Knowledge of clinical medicine and basic sciences.
- Technical, diagnostic and communication skills.
- Sound judgement in the application of knowledge and skills, demonstrating an awareness of personal limits of competence.

Being permitted to practice without *immediate supervision* is regarded as a key milestone in the training of a novice anaesthetist.

The RCA has highlighted the importance of this step by devising the 'Initial Assessment of Clinical Competency'. This highly structured and mandatory test is designed to confirm basic knowledge, ability in specific skills and a proper approach to patient care. For novice anaesthetists, the assessment is usually carried out after about 3 months of training. A doctor with previous anaesthetic experience from outside the UK is also required to take this test before working without immediate supervision. The test is in five parts:

- Preoperative assessment
- General anaesthesia for ASA 1 or 2 patients
- Rapid sequence induction
- Cardiopulmonary resuscitation skills
- Clinical judgement, attitudes and behaviour.

The clinical skills and knowledge expected for all the components of the test are outlined in the RCA training manual. The assessment must be carried out according to College instructions and is the responsibility of the College Tutor and involves at least two consultants.

Good professional practice means more than the sound application of clinical knowledge and skills. Assessment of *attitudes* is regarded as crucial at this very formative stage of training. The GMC have set out the standards of professional behaviour expected of doctors, and trainees should understand the importance of attitudes in professional practice including:

- Maintaining trust; respecting the views of the patient; respecting the right of the patient to dignity, privacy and confidentiality.
- Reliability; maintaining high levels of personal conduct; being dependable and conscientious in patient care.
- Maintaining good practice; demonstrating a commitment to self directed learning; using educational opportunities; demonstrating a commitment to standards.

APPRAISAL

The overall objective of appraisal is to help and encourage the trainee to reach and maintain a high standard of performance. Appraisal is not a process to check whether established targets have been met; that is assessment. However, as appraisal inevitably includes an analysis of performance it is difficult to separate it entirely from assessment. The opportunity for self-assessment is a valuable part of appraisal.

Appraisal is used to:

- Identify strengths in the trainee and the training scheme and build on these.
- Enable the trainee to feel encouraged by good performance.
- Identify any weaknesses in the trainee and the training scheme and plan to improve these aspects of performance.
- Allow the trainee to share confidentially information about the working and learning environment.

At the end of the appraisal both parties confirm areas of confidentiality, agree an outcome and produce documentation in the form of a summary sheet, an action plan and/or a personal learning plan.

PROFESSIONAL DEVELOPMENT

In addition to clinical training, personal and professional development are essential including the development of non-specialist skills.

Communication skills
Effective communication with patients involves more than verbal skills; establishing a rapport and learning to listen are just as important. Good communication includes the written word such as accurate records, patient summaries and referral letters. High standards of patient care also depend upon effective communication with colleagues, including non-medical team members.

Presentation skills
The ability to present information lucidly is a key non-specialist skill. The trainee should develop the necessary skills to present salient information succinctly both orally and in writing. At the basic level this involves presenting information about an individual patient to a colleague. New trainees also need to learn and practise the skills of formal presentation including case presentations at morbidity and mortality meetings, teaching sessions and journal club meetings.

Teaching skills
All doctors should contribute to a learning culture and the education of others.

Team working skills
Team working skills are necessary in order to establish effective working relationships with other colleagues and the multi-disciplinary team.

Management skills

At a junior level management skills include learning how to organize time and workload effectively. At a higher level the trainee learns to understand wider management issues, initially within their own department.

UNDERSTANDING MANAGEMENT ISSUES

Junior trainees need to develop an understanding of health service management in order to place their daily activities in context. Trainees should develop an understanding of the emphasis that is now placed upon the evaluation of medical care.

In order to achieve this, the trainee should understand and be involved with the areas described below.

Clinical governance

This refers to the quality of health care offered within an organization.

Clinical audit

Audit is the continual evaluation and measurement of how well the care that is provided meets the standards that have been set. Trainees must develop an understanding of clinical audit by progressing through the audit cycle.

Clinical risk management

This is the identification, analysis and control of circumstances or practices that put patients at risk.

Clinical effectiveness and evidence-based practice

The trainee should develop an understanding of evidence-based practice and assessment of clinical effectiveness. This requires a range of skills and facilities:

- Access to journals and libraries
- Information retrieval
- Sufficient knowledge of research to critically appraise papers
- Support from the organization to put evidence into practice.

Research

Junior trainees are not usually expected to undertake research projects but should develop an understanding of research including:

- Research methodology
- Ethical considerations
- Statistical analysis
- Critical appraisal of scientific papers
- Use of library resources and information searches using the internet and Medline.

THE PRIMARY EXAMINATION

The Primary FRCA Examination is an extensive and in-depth test of knowledge of basic sciences in addition to clinical knowledge and skills. The RCA website contains information about:

- Eligibility to sit the examination.
- The structure of the examination (see Table 18.2).
- Arrangements for the guidance of candidates who are unsuccessful.

TABLE 18.2 Structure of the Primary Examination

Examination section	Time allocated	Knowledge and skills tested
Multiple Choice Paper	3 hours	30 biochemistry and physiology questions 30 pharmacology questions 30 physics and clinical measurement questions
Objective Structured Clinical Examination (OSCE)	16 stations – 1 hour 40 min	Resuscitation and technical skills Anatomy and local anaesthetic blocks Skills in history taking and physical examination Communication skills Data interpretation Anaesthetic and monitoring equipment Anaesthetic hazards
Viva 1	15 min 15 min	Pharmacology Physiology and biochemistry
Viva 2	15 min 15 min	Physics, measurement, equipment and safety Clinical topics including a critical incident

The syllabus is contained within the RCA training manual. Individual study is a very important factor for success in the Primary Examination. Local College Tutors will assist in examination preparation and give candidates advice about suitable local and national courses.

REQUIREMENTS FOR ENTRY INTO THE SPECIALIST REGISTRAR GRADE/HIGHER SPECIALIST TRAINING

In the system in place at the time of writing the requirements to enter the Specialist Registrar (SpR) grade are:

- Full or limited registration with the GMC.
- At least 2 years training as an SHO in anaesthesia, of which one year must have been in a recognized training post in the UK.
- Completed at least 3 months training in Intensive Care Medicine.
- Passed the Primary FRCA Examination or an equivalent overseas exempting examination recognized by the RCA.
- Demonstrated satisfactory attitudes and behaviour.
- Been issued with an SHO Training Certificate to confirm satisfactory completion of SHO training.

When a College Tutor signs the SHO certificate, he or she is confirming that the trainers are satisfied that the trainee has obtained the competencies expected after two years of training, not merely that a time period has been completed. It is essential that there is evidence of satisfactory workplace assessments during the training period.

FURTHER READING

Comprehensive texts

Trainees should acquire a broad-based and comprehensive introductory text that will act as a basis for the Primary Examination.

Aitkenhead AR, Rowbotham D, and Smith G (2006) Textbook of Anaesthesia, 4th edn. Edinburgh: Churchill Livingstone.

Pinnock C, Smith T, and Lin E (2002) Fundamentals of Anaesthesia. London: Greenwich Medical Media.

Equipment textbook

Kenny G and Davis PD (2003) Basic Physics and Measurement in Anaesthesia. London: Butterworth-Heinemann.

Basic sciences

Trainees working towards the Primary FRCA Examination will need to refer to:

- General physiology text
- Anaesthetic pharmacology book
- Monographs on respiratory and cardiovascular physiology
- Anatomy textbook.

Non-clinical reading

General Medical Council Publications: 'Good Medical Practice' and 'The Early Years'.
www.gmc-uk.org/education/postgraduate/early_years.asp
www.gmc-uk.org/guidance/good_medical_practice/index.asp

Draper H and Scott WE (2004) Ethics in Anaesthesia and Intensive Care. London: Butterworth-Heinemann.

Greenhalgh T (2006) How to Read a Paper, 2nd edn. Oxford: Blackwell Publishing.

Roberts R (1999) Making Use of Information for Evidence-based Care. Oxford: Radcliffe Medical Press.

Web resources

Royal College of Anaesthetists: www.rcoa.ac.uk

Association of Anaesthetists of Great Britain and Ireland: www.aagbi.org.uk

Anaesthetic journals

British Journal of Anaesthesia. The journal of the Royal College of Anaesthetists. Oxford: Oxford University Press.

Anaesthesia. The journal of the Association of Anaesthetists of Great Britain and Ireland. Oxford: Blackwell Publishing.

ACTION PLANS

1. AIR EMBOLISM

Definition
A collection of air in the venous system

Clinical features
The air usually gets trapped in the right atrium or ventricle, forming a blockage to blood flow to the lungs.

Air may pass through a patent foramen ovale and embolize to the cerebral circulation.

Common in the sitting position (neurosurgery).

Common in the prone position (for example spinal surgery).

The early signs of air embolism include a sudden reduction in end-tidal carbon dioxide (due to increased deadspace), increased end-tidal nitrogen, and detection of emboli on echocardiography or precordial Doppler.

Late signs include increased central venous pressure, hypoxia, hypotension, shock and a continuous mill-wheel murmur.

Diagnosis
High index of suspicion during high-risk cases.

Echocardiography.

Increase in end-tidal nitrogen.

Management
Prevent further air entry (level patient out, flood wound with normal saline, and during neurosurgery compress the internal jugular veins).

Give 100% oxygen.

Position the patient in left lateral position to minimize the air lock.

Aspirate air from right atrium through a central venous catheter.

Supportive measures.

2. ADVANCED LIFE SUPPORT ALGORITHM

See Figure 19.1

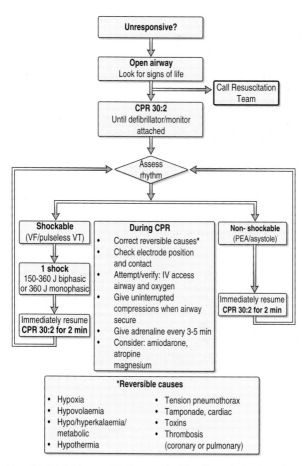

Fig. 19.1 Adult Advanced Life Support Algorithm. (Resuscitation Council, UK.)

3. ANAPHYLAXIS

Definition
A hypersensitivity reaction – anaphylactic or anaphylactoid (non IgE).

Clinical features
Shock, bronchospasm, pulmonary oedema, erythema, urticaria and oedema (including airway oedema), abdominal pain (if awake).

Diagnosis
High index of suspicion with use of known allergens.
Clinical features may be indistinguishable from other forms of shock.
Definitive diagnosis may depend on demonstration of elevated plasma tryptase levels.

Action
Stop administration of drug (or other allergen).
Establish airway.
Intermittent positive pressure ventilation with 100% oxygen.
Establish wide-bore intravenous access.
Adrenaline (epinephrine):

- 50–100 μg intravenously, repeat as necessary (0.5–1 ml of 1:10,000 solution).
- Alternatively, 0.5–1.0 mg intramuscularly, if no i.v. access.

Volume expansion with colloid or crystalloid.
Adrenaline (epinephrine) or noradrenaline (norepinephrine) infusion for persistent hypotension.

 Colloid may be the cause of the anaphylaxis.

Secondary therapy
Sodium bicarbonate for metabolic acidosis.
Antihistamine – chlorpheniramine 10–20 mg by slow intravenous injection.
Corticosteroids – hydrocortisone 100 mg intravenously.
Bronchodilators (aminophylline or volatile anaesthetics) for persistent bronchospasm.
Take blood (10 ml in plain bottle) for plasma tryptase measurement at 1 hour.
Arrange immunology referral for skin patch testing

4. BRONCHOSPASM

Definition
Constriction of airways due to muscular constriction and oedema, often associated with increased secretions.

Clinical features
More likely in patients with chronic obstructive pulmonary disease, asthma or smoking.

Can occur with or without a history of asthma especially with a recent upper airway infection, following carinal or bronchial stimulation with a tracheal tube during light anaesthesia, during bronchoscopy/mediastinoscopy, with beta-blockers.

Leads to inadequate tidal volume; increased work of breathing; hypoxia and later hypercarbia; difficulty in IPPV; increased airway pressure during inspiration; barotrauma to lungs and pneumothorax; and inability to clear airway secretions.

May be associated with anaphylaxis and histamine releasing drugs (such as atracurium).

Diagnosis
High airway pressures during IPPV.

Wheeze may be absent in tight bronchospasm.

Exclude other causes of high airway pressure or wheeze – mechanical obstruction, pneumothorax, pulmonary oedema.

Bronchospasm associated with cardiovascular collapse suggests a severe allergic reaction or anaphylaxis.

Action
Treat hypoxia with oxygen 100%.

Remove the stimulus (e.g. reposition tracheal tube if too long).

Intraoperative wheeze – deepen anaesthesia, ensure adequate analgesia. (Inhaled anaesthetics are all bronchodilators).

Salbutamol, nebulized 5 mg or intravenous infusion – 3 µg/kg by slow bolus followed by infusion (watch for tachycardia and hypokalaemia); presence of hypoxia or hypercarbia increases the risk of arrhythmias.

Intravenous aminophylline 5 mg/kg, slowly, followed by an infusion (toxicity is possible if patient already on theophyllines).

Epinephrine if anaphylaxis or severe allergic reaction is suspected.

Hydrocortisone 100 mg.

If these measures fail: paralyse and ventilate (if not already), maintain peak airway pressures <30 mmHg, permit hypercapnia in preference to high airway pressure, allow adequate expiratory time to prevent air trapping, postpone surgery and arrange ICU admission.

5. CARDIAC TAMPONADE

Definition
An accumulation of fluid in the pericardial cavity.

Clinical features
Increased pressure in the pericardial cavity leads to a reduction in ventricular filling and consequently a reduction in cardiac output and hypotension.

Rapid accumulation of fluid can lead to collapse within minutes.

Causes: chest trauma, cardiac surgery, pericarditis (viral, pyogenic, uraemic or post-radiation), myocardial perforation with central venous catheters and pulmonary artery catheters, aortic dissection.

As well as shock, there may be jugular venous distension, muffled heart sounds, a low voltage ECG, pulsus paradoxus (low pulse volume during inspiration), Kussmaul's sign (distension of jugular veins during inspiration).

Diagnosis
High index of suspicion – especially in penetrating chest trauma.

Enlarged heart on chest X-ray.

Echocardiography.

Treatment
Pericardial drainage of blood or other fluid through a long needle (22 G spinal needle) inserted between the xiphisternum and left costal margin, directed towards the left shoulder. Complications include pneumothorax, myocardial rupture and coronary artery laceration. Supportive measures including intravenous fluids and vasopressors. Prevent further accumulation (a drain can be left in place); urgent surgery if tamponade is due to trauma.

6. CHRONIC ANAEMIA

Definition
Long-standing anaemia, that is usually, at least partially, compensated for by the body.

Clinical features
Many possible causes including lack of haematinics (e.g. iron deficiency, or vitamin B_{12} deficiency), chronic disease (e.g. rheumatoid arthritis), chronic renal impairment, and drug reactions.
Chronic active bleeding such as peptic ulceration or large bowel tumours lead to progressive iron deficiency anaemia.
Patients are usually well compensated by an increase in plasma volume.
Complications include worsening angina, breathlessness, marked lethargy, faints or falls.
Cardiovascular changes such as tachycardia suggest a more acute cause.

Diagnosis
Measurement of the haemoglobin concentration. The usual lower limit is 11.5 g/dl for women and 13.5 g/dl men. However, each laboratory has its own reference value for the lower limit of normal.

Action
Newly diagnosed mild anaemia, or patients undergoing minor surgery with little risk of blood loss can proceed with surgery and be investigated afterwards.
Patients with more severe anaemia, especially if associated with complications or patients undergoing major elective surgery need investigating preoperatively.
In urgent or emergency cases proceed with cross-matched blood available.
Mild-to-moderate anaemia of known aetiology that is well-compensated does not need treating.
Patients with severe anaemia secondary to chronic disease may be treated with erythropoetin prior to surgery.

7. CHRONIC RENAL FAILURE

Definition
A long-standing impairment of renal function.

Clinical features
Severity of effects depends on the degree of impairment.
Effects usually only seen when renal function is reduced by more than 50%.
Leads to problems with fluid balance (usually overload, but can be dehydration in polyuric renal failure).
Electrolyte and acid–base disturbance – especially hyperkalaemia.
May produce anaemia and hypertension.

Diagnosis
Measure urea and electrolytes preoperatively in all patients with established renal impairment, the elderly (>60), those with long-term severe co-morbidity, and those undergoing major surgery.

Action
For patients on haemodialysis, undertake surgery just after dialysis to ensure the best metabolic and electrolyte control.
Ensure hypertension is adequately controlled.
Avoid NSAIDs.
Avoid renally-excreted drugs including those with renally excreted active metabolites such as morphine.
Atracurium is the safest muscle relaxant.
Avoid placing cannulae in limbs containing a shunt or fistula.
Induction of anaesthesia may be associated with marked hypotension, and patients may require infusion of intravenous fluid to overcome this.
Fluid balance for major cases may require use of central venous pressure monitoring.
Suxamethonium is safe to use if the baseline potassium level is normal (the rise with suxamethonium is not exaggerated).

8. DIABETES MELLITUS

Definition
Abnormal glucose metabolism and homeostasis.
Differentiated into insulin-dependent (IDDM) and non-insulin
dependent (NIDDM). Insulin-dependent diabetics must always
receive insulin and glucose to prevent catabolism and ketoacidosis.

Clinical features
IDDM patients are usually thin, and require regular insulin.
NIDDM patients are usually overweight; controlled either with
diet, oral hypoglycaemics or insulin (insulin-requiring).
Increased incidence of atherosclerotic disease, renal impairment,
and neuropathies including autonomic neuropathies leading to
cardiovascular instability and gastroparesis.
Increased risk of postoperative infection.

Action
Assess preoperative diabetic control.
Anaesthesia/surgery should be delayed (if possible) if control is
poor. Patients requiring emergency surgery may have developed
diabetic ketoacidosis and require resuscitation. These patients
require specialist help in management of the severe dehydration
and metabolic disturbance.
If possible diabetics should be first on the morning list.

NIDDM:
Patients can usually withstand short periods of starvation without
treatment. They may need insulin if undergoing prolonged or
major surgery, or if their diabetes becomes uncontrolled following
minor surgery.
Stop oral hypoglycaemics the day before surgery (chlorpropamide
at least 48 hours before).

IDDM:
Patients require insulin when starved and throughout the periop-
erative period.
Do not give long-acting insulin the night before surgery.
Stop all subcutaneous insulin on day of surgery, monitor blood
glucose every hour for 4 hours and then 2 hourly.
Start insulin/glucose therapy:

- Use a variable-rate insulin infusion (soluble insulin 50 i.u. in
  50 ml normal saline by syringe driver) and adjust rate as required

(usually start at 1–2 units per hour). Ensure patient is always receiving some carbohydrate, *or*

- Use the Alberti regime (not suitable if poorly controlled or prolonged therapy needed). Glucose 10% 500 ml; human soluble insulin 10 i.u.; KCl 10 mmol. Infuse over 5 hours via a dedicated cannula. Adjust insulin and KCl concentrations according to results.

  Aim for a blood glucose of 6–10 mmol/L

Normal management regimes can be restarted when normal oral food intake has resumed.

9. DRUG OR ALCOHOL ADDICTION

Definition

Consumption of drugs or alcohol associated with physical or psychological dependency, or both.

Clinical features

Alcohol

Drug metabolizing enzymes are induced leading to tolerance to anaesthetic agents and other sedatives.

Associated with liver damage and cirrhosis, cardiomyopathy, pancreatitis, nutritional and vitamin deficiencies, cerebral degeneration.

Acute withdrawal leads to delirium tremens (DTs) – disorientation, hallucinations, increased psychomotor activity and increased autonomic activity lasting up to 10 days.

Drugs

Intravenous drug abuse leads to thrombophlebitis, abscesses, sepsis, and HIV infection.

Narcotic abuse leads to resistance to sedatives and anaesthetic agents. Withdrawal symptoms include cramps, vomiting and diarrhoea.

Cannabis use may be associated with tachycardia and hypertension.

Cocaine use may produce myocardial ischaemia and cardiomyopathy.

Amphetamine use increases requirements of anaesthetic agents (including an increase in MAC).

Action

Central venous access may be required in intravenous drug abusers.

Alcoholics should be given vitamins – in particular thiamine.

Pre-empt DTs with sedatives, e.g. oral chlordiazepoxide; re-establish some consumption of alcohol postoperatively if it safe to do so.

The rate of spontaneous ventilation may assist titration of opioid analgesia in narcotic abusers.

Involve local alcohol and drug abuse teams.

10. FAILED INTUBATION AND DIFFICULT INTUBATION ALGORITHMS

Definition
Failure to position a tube correctly in the upper trachea, with the cuff inflated (adults), and secured in place in patients in whom difficulty with intubation was not predicted.

Clinical features
Risk is up to 1 in 300 in obstetric anaesthesia or during rapid sequence induction, less in non-pregnant population.
Usually due to a poor view of the laryngeal inlet at laryngoscopy.
Failure may be due to a lack of time to complete intubation before desaturation starts.

Diagnosis
Failure to see tracheal tube pass between vocal cords.
Absence of carbon dioxide waveform on capnography.

Action
Call for help immediately.
Determine if it is possible to ventilate the patient:

- If mask ventilation is possible – then follow non-emergency pathway (Can ventilate, can't intubate). See Figures 19.2 & 19.3.
- If ventilation with face-mask is not possible – then follow emergency pathway (Can't ventilate, can't intubate). See Figure 19.4.

If surgery is not urgent the best course of action if intubation is not possible is to wake the patient.
Once oxygenation is established await return of spontaneous ventilation and wait for the patient to wake up.
If surgery is urgent because the patient's life is in danger, it may be necessary to continue with whatever 'airway' is achieved.
If there is no risk of regurgitation and aspiration, and the achieved airway is satisfactory, surgery may continue.
The timing and place of emergence should be considered and suitable help should be available.

Non-emergency pathway (Can ventilate, can't intubate)
Try:

- Different laryngoscopes and blades
- Different bougies
- Laryngeal mask airway-guided intubation

- Fibreoptic intubation
- Laryngeal mask airway
- Surgical tracheostomy.

Emergency pathway (Can't ventilate, can't intubate)
Try:

- Manoeuvres such as repositioning, different oral or nasal airways
- Different laryngeal mask airways (including iLMA, and ProSeal LMA)
- Needle cricothyroidotomy and jet ventilation
- Surgical cricothyroidotomy
- Percutaneous cricothyroidotomy kits
- Jet ventilation through rigid bronchoscope
- Oesophageal-tracheal Combitube.

Maintain cricoid pressure in patients at risk of regurgitation if possible, but ensure oxygenation (with release of cricoid pressure if necessary).

Please refer to the Difficult Airway Society algorithms below (Figures 19.2–19.4). Guidelines from the Difficult Airway Society are available: Henderson JJ, Popat MT, Latto IP, Pearce AC. Difficult Airway Society guidelines for management of the unanticipated difficult intubation. Anaesthesia 2004; 59:675–694.

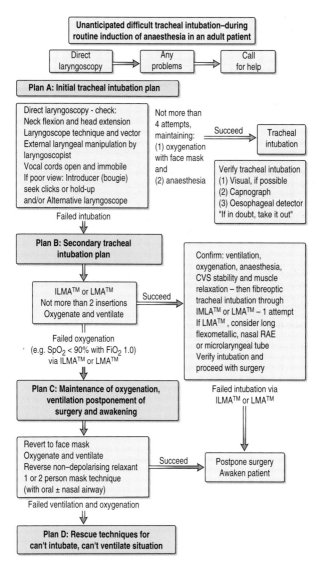

Fig. 19.2 Unanticipated difficult tracheal intubation – during routine induction of anaesthesia in an adult patient. (Adapted from Difficult Airway Society Guidelines.)

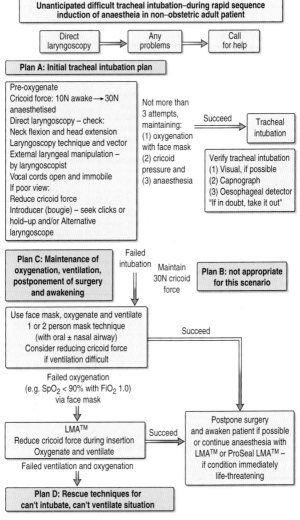

Fig. 19.3 Unanticipated difficult tracheal intubation – during rapid sequence induction of anaesthesia in non-obstetric adult patient. (Adapted from Difficult Airway Society Guidelines.)

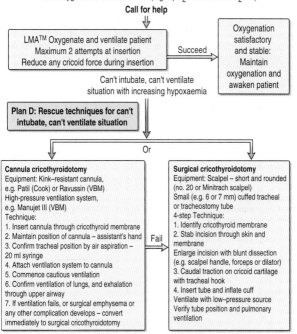

**Failed intubation, increasing hypoxaemia and difficult ventilation
in the paralysed anaesthetized patient:
Rescue techniques for the can't intubate, can't ventilate situation**

Failed intubation and difficult ventilation (other than laryngospasm)

Face mask
Oxygenate and ventilate patient
Maximum head extension
Maximum jaw thrust
Assistance with mask seal
Oral ± 6mm nasal airway
Reduce cricoid force - if necessary

Failed oxygenation with face mask (e.g. SpO₂ < 90% with FiO₂ 1.0)

Call for help

LMA™ Oxygenate and ventilate patient
Maximum 2 attempts at insertion
Reduce any cricoid force during insertion

Succeed →

Oxygenation
satisfactory
and stable:
Maintain
oxygenation and
awaken patient

Can't intubate, can't ventilate
situation with increasing hypoxaemia

**Plan D: Rescue techniques for can't
intubate, can't ventilate situation**

Or

Cannula cricothyroidotomy
Equipment: Kink–resistant cannula,
e.g. Patil (Cook) or Ravussin (VBM)
High-pressure ventilation system,
e.g. Manujet III (VBM)
Technique:
1. Insert cannula through cricothyroid membrane
2. Maintain position of cannula – assistant's hand
3. Confirm tracheal position by air aspiration –
20 ml syringe
4. Attach ventilation system to cannula
5. Commence cautious ventilation
6. Confirm ventilation of lungs, and exhalation
through upper airway
7. If ventilation fails, or surgical emphysema or
any other complication develops – convert
immediately to surgical cricothyroidotomy

Fail →

Surgical cricothyroidotomy
Equipment: Scalpel – short and rounded
(no. 20 or Minitrach scalpel)
Small (e.g. 6 or 7 mm) cuffed tracheal
or tracheostomy tube
4-step Technique:
1. Identify cricothyroid membrane
2. Stab incision through skin and
membrane
Enlarge incision with blunt dissection
(e.g. scalpel handle, forceps or dilator)
3. Caudal traction on cricoid cartilage
with tracheal hook
4. Insert tube and inflate cuff
Ventilate with low–pressure source
Verify tube position and pulmonary
ventilation

Notes:
1. These techniques can have serious complications – use only in life-threatening situations
2. Convert to definitive airway as soon as possible
3. Postoperative management – see other difficult airway guidelines and flow–charts
4. 4 mm cannula with low–pressure ventilation may be successful in patient breathing spontaneously

Fig. 19.4 Failed intubation, increasing hypoxaemia and difficult ventilation in
the paralysed anaesthetized patient: rescue techniques for the 'can't intubate,
can't ventilate' situation. (Adapted from Difficult Airway Society Guidelines.)

11. FAILURE TO RECOVER AFTER GENERAL ANAESTHESIA

Definition
Failure to recover from anaesthesia within the expected time period (usually 5–10 min after stopping anaesthesia).

Clinical features
Most common in the elderly.

Usually associated with inadvertent anaesthetic drug overdosage or persistent neuromuscular blockade.

May be a sign of intraoperative catastrophe such as cerebrovascular accident.

Metabolism of drugs may be reduced in the elderly, hypothermic, hypothyroid, and patients with abnormal hepatic or renal function.

Consider central cholinergic syndrome following use of anticholinergic agents in the elderly.

Diagnosis
Assess pupils – small and equal suggests still anaesthetized or too much opioid.

Assess neuromuscular function with nerve stimulator – fade suggests continuing non-depolarizing block; consider suxamethonium apnoea if this drug was used. If either a possibility ensure patient is not aware. Need to exclude:

- hypoglycaemia (especially if diabetic and on insulin regime)
- hypoxaemia
- hypercapnia
- hypotension
- TURP syndrome after TURP surgery.

Full neurological examination to exclude cerebrovascular accident or post-ictal state and consider CT scan.

Action
Correct any abnormality, if found.

If due to persistent non-depolarizing block, repeat the anticholinesterase drug.

Central cholinergic syndrome can be treated with physostigmine.

Await metabolism of sedative or hypnotic drugs.

12. HYPERCARBIA

Definition
A rise in arterial carbon dioxide tension to a level greater than that expected for the clinical state.
(An exact definition is not possible because the 'normal' upper limit depends on the depth of anaesthesia.)

Clinical features
Either due to increased production of carbon dioxide or inadequate ventilation.
It is quite common intraoperatively during spontaneous breathing and in the postoperative period when patients are receiving opioids.
Causes: central depressants (general anaesthetics, benzodiazepines, opioids); neuromuscular depression; increased airway resistance (bronchospasm, obstruction); rebreathing; increased carbon dioxide 'production' (laparoscopy, hyperthyroidism, malignant hyperthermia).
May cause cardiovascular stimulation (followed by depression at greater concentrations).

Diagnosis
Precise diagnosis needs arterial blood gases. End-tidal carbon dioxide concentration may be used as an alternative.
A persistent or continual rise may suggest malignant hyperthermia (see Action Plan 23).

Action
Find the cause.
Mild hypercarbia does not need treatment.
Progressive hypercarbia or if associated with cardiovascular changes requires controlled ventilation to correct.

13. HYPERTENSION – PERIOPERATIVE

Definition
The normal maximum level depends on age.
An alternative definition during or after anaesthesia is a sustained increase of 20% or more from baseline (preoperative) level.

Clinical features
Myocardial ischaemia.
Cerebrovascular accident.
Increased intraoperative bleeding.
Causes: light anaesthesia; pain; essential hypertension; Cushing's response to raised intracranial pressure; undiagnosed phaeochromocytoma, thyroid storm, sudden increase in afterload – e.g. aortic cross clamping; hypercapnia; malignant hyperthermia, laryngoscopy.

Diagnosis
Non-invasive automated blood pressure. Check the cuff is correct size and tubing not kinked.
If the diagnosis is in doubt or precise control of blood pressure is needed consider use of an intra-arterial cannula for direct measurement.

Action
Find cause and *always* consider possibility of light anaesthesia or awareness.
Antihypertensives: vasodilators (hydralazine [2.5 mg bolus]), GTN (infusion), sodium nitroprusside (infusion); beta-blockers: (esmolol [bolus and infusion], labetalol [5–10 mg bolus]).

 Never use an antihypertensive to control intraoperative hypertension unless you are sure the patient is not aware or in pain.

14. HYPOTENSION – PERIOPERATIVE

Definition
MAP less than 60 mmHg (this lower limit is higher in patients with pre-existing hypertension), or a sustained fall of more than 20% from the preoperative (baseline) level.

Clinical features
Associated with tissue hypoperfusion and organ ischaemia – in particular the myocardium, brain, kidney and gut.

Possible causes: hypovolaemia – preoperative dehydration, losses during surgery – blood, evaporative (e.g. from open abdomen), sequestration into tissues; relative hypovolaemia secondary to sympathetic block (central neuraxis blockade with local anaesthetics); decreased venous return – PE, secondary to positive-pressure ventilation, aortocaval compression by gravid uterus; overdosage of anaesthetic drugs; arrhythmias; or shock (anaphylaxis, cardiogenic shock, pneumothorax, tamponade, septic).

The commonest postoperative causes are usually hypovolaemia or the effects of residual anaesthetic agents.

Diagnosis
Non-invasive automated blood pressure machine. Check cuff and tubing.

If diagnosis in doubt consider use of arterial cannula for direct blood pressure measurement.

Action
Assume hypovolaemia until proved otherwise and infuse fluid (crystalloid/colloid/blood according to type of fluid lost).

Estimate recent losses, otherwise try fluid bolus, e.g. 10 ml/kg of crystalloid or 250–500 ml colloid, and assess response.

If no response, repeat fluid challenge and consider other causes or ongoing fluid loss.

Reduce anaesthesia depth but avoid awareness.

Investigate for other causes of hypotension and treat as appropriate. Increase inspired concentration of oxygen.

Boluses of either a vasoconstrictor (methoxamine, 1–5 mg; metaraminol, 0.5–1 mg; phenylephrine 0.1–0.2 mg) or a sympathetomimetic (ephedrine, 3 mg boluses), or *in extremis,* epinephrine 0.05–0.1 mg, should be used for vasodilatation (e.g. after sympathetic block, anaphylaxis or sepsis) and should *not* be used to manage hypovolaemia. A continuous infusion may be required for persistent hypotension.

15. HYPERTHERMIA

Definition
A core temperature >38°C.

Clinical features
Rare intraoperatively.
Possible causes:
malignant hyperthermia (see Action Plan 23);
inflammation (intraoperatively only during major surgery, more
common postoperatively);
increased metabolic state due to thyrotoxicosis;
hypothalamic injury (particularly head injury);
neurolept malignant syndrome;
use of sympathomimetics – MAO inhibitors, amphetamines,
cocaine and tricylcic antidepressants;
use of atropine which reduces sweating.

An increase in temperature may lead to increased oxygen requirement, tissue hypoxia, increased glucose demand, increased carbon
dioxide production and metabolic acidosis.

Diagnosis
Temperature monitoring.

Treatment
Eliminate the cause.
Malignant hyperthermia – see Action Plan 23.
Maintain oxygenation and cardiovascular stability.
Reduce ambient temperature if possible.
Cooling blankets.
Vasodilatation such as chlorpromazine.
In extreme cases, internal lavage of the bladder (using a urinary
catheter), stomach (using a nasogastric tube) or peritoneum (if the
abdomen is already open) should be performed with cold normal
saline.

16. HYPOTHERMIA

Definition
Core temperature <35°C.

Clinical features
Heat loss due to radiation, evaporation and convection.
Use of cold fluids intravenously or for lavage.
Risk factors include the elderly, prolonged procedures, open body cavities and extensive burns.
May lead to delayed emergence, slower drug metabolism, metabolic acidosis, arrhythmias, coagulopathy.
Shivering leads to increased oxygen requirement, discomfort, and muscle spasms.

Diagnosis
Temperature measurement.

Action
Prevention.
Cover exposed body surfaces.
Forced warm air blankets.
Warm all intravenous fluids.
Use closed-circuit technique.
Warming blankets underneath patient.
(Extracorporeal circulation is required for cardiac arrest secondary to severe hypothermia, for example immersion hypothermia.)

17. HYPOXAEMIA

Definition
A reduction (<90%) in the oxygen saturation of haemoglobin in the peripheral blood.

Clinical features
A fall in peripheral blood oxygen saturation results in a reduction in oxygen delivery to the tissues.
Leads to tissue hypoxia and organ ischaemia.
May lead to organ failure – e.g. shock, confusion.

Diagnosis
A reduction in peripheral blood oxygen saturation as detected by pulse oximeter.
Ensure that the oximeter reading is correct (a false reading can result from reduced peripheral perfusion from shock, cold extremities, peripheral limb movements, high ambient light). If in doubt check arterial blood gases.
Cyanosis is an unreliable sign.

Action
Look for causes and treat as appropriate:
Reduction in saturation of central blood:
Low oxygen concentration in anaesthetic circuit
Inadequate ventilation of lungs (ventilator failure, airway obstruction)
Abnormal lung function (for example – collapse, pneumothorax)
Reduced blood flow to lungs – shock, pulmonary embolism.

Reduced blood flow to peripheries:
Shock.

Increase inspired oxygen concentration (100%)
Ensure adequate ventilation by manually 'bagging' the patient's lungs
Assess pulse and cardiac output
Chest X-ray if diagnosis unsure.

18. INTRAOPERATIVE MYOCARDIAL ISCHAEMIA

Definition
An abnormality of blood flow to the myocardium leading to a myocardial oxygen supply less than the metabolic demand requires.

Clinical features
May be associated with increased demand (tachycardia, hypertension) or reduced supply (hypotension, hypovolaemia).
Electrocardiographic changes *may* be seen (ST depression, T wave inversion, ST elevation, arrhythmias).
If awake may have angina or may be asymptomatic (silent ischaemia).
Intraoperative myocardial ischaemia may present as arrhythmias, hypotension, organ hypoperfusion, myocardial infarction, or cardiac arrest.
Perioperative myocardial infarction has a greater mortality than infarction at other times.

Diagnosis
Presence of angina.
12-lead ECG. Intraoperative ischaemia may not be detected by standard 'three-lead' ECG.
Diagnosis of exclusion in low cardiac output state.
Rise in 'cardiac enzymes'.
Echocardiography showing new regional wall motion abnormalities.

Action
Correct precipitating cause.
Increase inspired oxygen concentration.
Decrease cardiac load with beta-blockers (e.g. esmolol, 0.5–1 mg/kg) or GTN infusion.
Inotropic support for persistent low cardiac output state.
For persistent ischaemia or possible infarction: cardiac enzyme analysis; treat as for acute coronary syndrome; arrange HDU, ICU or CCU admission; and start aspirin if not contraindicated by surgery.
Thrombolytics usually contraindicated during after surgery.

19. JEHOVAH'S WITNESSES

Definition
A branch of Christianity in which the believers do not agree to transfusion of blood products (among other beliefs).

Features
Believers refuse blood or any blood product which has been outside the body. There may be different interpretations of this belief, with individual followers guided by a local committee of senior figures.
Some Jehovah's Witnesses will accept blood that has been in a cell-saver, or a cardiac bypass machine – as this blood is still in contiguity with blood in the body.
Most will not accept autologous blood (such as from pre-donation).

Action
Believers are asked to sign a different consent form where they can declare their wish not to receive blood.
Anaesthetists should ensure that the patient is aware of the risks and that their decision is 'informed'.
Measure haemoglobin concentration preoperatively.
Consider erythropoetin to increase preoperative haemoglobin if the patient agrees.
Plan to use cell-saver technology in cases at risk of bleeding intra-operatively, providing the patient agrees.
Replace blood loss with crystalloid or colloid (not plasma!).
Practitioners must not give blood (or any other treatment) to a competent individual who has elected not to receive that product (or treatment), even if not giving such products is likely to lead to the death of the patient.
An application can be made to the Court to treat children of believers below the age of being able to give their own consent (Gillick incompetent). Practitioners MUST take advice from senior colleagues and their institution's legal advisors beforehand.
In *extremis* practitioners may treat children unable to give their own consent (Gillick incompetent) with blood if, in the practitioner's opinion, it is life-saving at that moment and there is no time to consult the Court.

20. LARYNGOSPASM

Definition
Spasm of the laryngeal muscles causing partial or complete obstruction to airflow.

Clinical features
Usually caused by irritation of the airway during light anaesthesia. Precipitating factors include insertion of an oropharyngeal airway or laryngeal mask airway; oral secretions; blood or vomitus in the mouth; pungent volatile anaesthetic; laryngoscopy; or painful stimulus during light anaesthesia such as peritoneal traction, anal stretch, or movement of a fractured limb.

Results in stridor, suprasternal and supraclavicular recession and paradoxical respiratory movements (during inspiration the abdomen rises and the chest retracts).

Persistent laryngospasm can cause hypoxia, hypercarbia and acidosis.

Diagnosis
Inspiratory stridor may help differentiate laryngospasm from bronchospasm and upper airway obstruction.

Action
Remove the stimulus.

Intraoperatively deepen anaesthesia; postoperatively continue to lighten (unless suxamethonium used – see below).

Give 100% oxygen.

Continuous positive airway pressure of up to $20\,cmH_2O$ with a tight mask fitting until the laryngeal spasm breaks (use a normal mask and a partially closed expiratory (spill) valve), decompress the airway occasionally (by removing the mask from the face).

Postoperatively spontaneous breathing will usually commence.

If breathing doesn't start, or for intraoperative laryngospasm, use gentle positive pressure ventilation.

In severe hypoxia and no sign of spontaneous recovery, suxamethonium should be given to break the spasm. This should be followed by 100% oxygen and deepening of anaesthesia before the noxious stimulus is resumed (at induction or intraoperatively), or to prevent awareness if laryngeal spasm occurs during emergence.

21. LOCAL ANAESTHETIC TOXICITY

Definition
Central nervous system or cardiovascular changes due to excess systemic concentrations of local anaesthetic.

Clinical features
Occurrence depends on total dose and route of administration; the fastest absorption occurs with intercostal blocks and epidural administration.
CNS effects are seen before CVS effects.
CNS stimulation followed by depression: restlessness, anxiety, tremor, convulsions.
CVS: hypotension, bradycardia, sweating, arrhythmias, cardiac arrest.
Allergic reactions are very rare with amide local anaesthetics, but more common with ester compounds.

Diagnosis
A high index of suspicion after use of local anaesthetics.
Measurement of blood concentration is not normally required.

Action
'ABC' management to maintain oxygenation and circulation.
Treat convulsions with small doses of benzodiazepines, e.g. diazepam.
Adrenergic agents to support cardiovascular system.
Intravenously administered Intralipid (a constituent of total parenteral nutrition) may bind local anaesthetic and may be used in cardiac arrest unresponsive to attempts at resuscitation.

22. MASSIVE TRANSFUSION

Definition
Replacement of total blood volume in 24 h or less or replacement of 20% of total blood volume in 1 h.

Clinical features
Infusion of stored blood leads to loss of clotting factors (particularly factors V and VIII) and platelet numbers and function. Complications include:

- disseminated intravascular coagulation
- hypothermia
- hypocalcaemia
- hyperkalaemia.

Diagnosis
Total blood volume is approximately 70–75 ml/kg in adults. Measuring blood loss in theatre is notoriously inaccurate. In patients at risk there should be frequent assessment of haemoglobin, platelet count, PT and partial thromboplastin time, and fibrinogen levels. Measure calcium and potassium levels.

Action
Warm all fluid to be infused (and maintain patient temperature with forced warm air blower).
Discuss the case with Haematologists and the haematology laboratory staff as early as possible.
Do not aim to transfuse to a 'normal' haemoglobin concentration. For most patients aim for around 9 g/dl.
In cases of massive sudden bleeding, e.g. trauma, when the blood group is not known, it may be necessary to start the transfusion with group O, Rh negative blood. Type specific blood is available within a few minutes, and cross-matched blood within about 40 min.
FFP (one unit per four units of blood), and platelets may be required to prevent/correct coagulopathies.
Cryoprecipitate may be required to maintain fibrinogen levels.
Keep accurate records of all transfused blood products.
Calcium may be required to maintain plasma calcium levels and counteract hyperkalaemia effects on the heart.

23. MALIGNANT HYPERTHERMIA

Definition
A hypermetabolic state that occurs in genetically susceptible patients on exposure to a triggering agent.

Clinical features
Core temperature increases by 2°C per hour or more, or 0.5°C every 15 min.

Triggers are the volatile anaesthetic agents and suxamethonium.

On exposure to a triggering agent patients undergo a sustained muscular contraction.

Failure to relax after suxamethonium.

The first sign may be masseter muscle spasm or inability to open the mouth after giving suxamethonium; however, not all masseter spasms progress to malignant hyperthermia.

Tachycardia, cardiac arrhythmias and cardiovascular collapse.

Increased end-tidal carbon dioxide and tachypnoea if the patient is breathing spontaneously.

Metabolic and respiratory acidosis.

Generalized muscular rigidity.

Hyperkalaemia.

Myoglobinurea causing acute tubular necrosis.

Previously uneventful general anaesthesia or exposure to triggers does not rule out the diagnosis.

Diagnosis
Definitive diagnosis is usually made after the event by muscle biopsy and in vitro testing in a specialist centre.

Action
Discontinue the triggering agent and end surgery if possible.

Give 100% oxygen.

Change the anaesthetic machine to a vapour-free machine.

Maintain anaesthesia with an alternative agent e.g. propofol.

Dantrolene 1–2 mg/kg i.v. should be given, and repeated every 5 min, until the temperature and carbon dioxide stop rising, up to a total of 10 mg/kg.

Treat acidosis with sodium bicarbonate 8.4%.

Treat hyperkalaemia with insulin and glucose.

Lower temperature by:

● body surface cooling
● cooling blankets

- cool irrigation fluids
- extracorporeal cooling may be indicated.

Maintain urine output >1 ml/kg/h.
Admit the patient to ICU for supportive therapy, prevention of secondary complications and close monitoring for recurrence.
Arrange muscle biopsy testing of patient (and near relatives if diagnosis confirmed).

Anaesthesia in patients with malignant hyperthermia susceptibility
Ensure dantrolene is available.
Use a vapour-free anaesthetic machine, flushed with 100% oxygen for 5 minutes at a fresh gas flow rate of 10 litres/minute.
All circuits should be disposable and new.
The soda lime should be previously unused.
Regional anaesthesia is safe.
Drugs which are considered safe include barbiturates, narcotics, nitrous oxide, propofol, benzodiazepines, non-depolarizing neuro-muscular blocking agents.
A total intravenous technique using propofol along with an infusion of short-acting opioids is safest.

24. OLIGURIA

Definition
Definition of oliguria is age-dependent.
In adults it is a urine output less than 0.5 ml/kg/h.

Clinical features
Oliguria is often a sign of an underlying problem such as hypovo-
laemia.
Oliguria (like renal failure) can be pre-renal, renal or postrenal.
The commonest cause in the perioperative period is pre-renal.
New-onset renal failure is rare in the perioperative period but could
be due to surgical damage, toxic effect of drugs, e.g. antibiotics, or
following myoglobinaemia in trauma patients.
Post-renal causes are due to obstruction – usually urinary retention
due to pain, drugs (e.g. opioids) or prostatic enlargement.

Diagnosis
Oliguria is first confirmed by excluding urinary retention.
If a catheter is in place its patency must be ensured.
Examine for hypovolaemia.

Action

Hypovolaemia
Correct hypovolaemia.
Consider fluid balance up to that point and correct any fluid
deficits as found.
Fluid bolus, e.g. 10 ml/kg of crystalloid over 10–15 min – the urine
output may increase and stay increased, output may increase tem-
porarily and then decrease again in which case ongoing hypovolaemia should be suspected, or output may not increase at all in which
case repeat the fluid bolus and reconsider diagnosis.
If oliguria is persistent or recurs, or in elderly patients or patients
with significant co-morbidity, consider central venous pressure
monitoring to assist fluid balance.
If oliguria persists despite adequate fluid loading and no obvious
cause of obstruction consider renal ultrasound.
Never treat oliguria with diuretics.

25. POST-DURAL PUNCTURE HEADACHE

Definition
Persistent and debilitating headache after dural puncture.

Clinical features
Rare (<1%) after subarachnoid anaesthesia.
Common after accidental dural puncture from a Tuohy needle.
Headache may be severe and debilitating.
Onset may be up to 5 days after dural puncture; it may persist for 6 weeks.
It is more common in young patients.
It is usually worse in the occipital regions and often associated with neck pain, but may be frontal and associated with orbital pain. It is worse on sitting.

Diagnosis
History of recent subarachnoid blockade or epidural catheter placement.

Action
Treatment with simple analgesics and encouragement of oral fluids or use of intravenous fluids may be sufficient.
Persistent or severe headache should be treated by an epidural 'blood patch'.

Epidural blood patch
Use full aseptic precautions for venepuncture and injection (two operators).
Take 20 ml of patient's own blood.
Inject 10–15 ml of blood into the epidural space at the same level as the previous puncture.
Stop injection if discomfort is reported.
Send the rest of the blood for culture.
May be repeated if unsuccessful.

26. PNEUMOTHORAX

Definition
A collection of air (occasionally other gas) in between the pleura, causing the lung to collapse (partially or completely).

Clinical features
Pneumothorax may occur as a result of trauma to the lung or chest wall, or during surgery such as oesophagoscopy.

Can occur following central venous cannulation or brachial plexus blockade, or as a result of ventilation in patients with emphysema or bullae.

A large pneumothorax can be associated with lung collapse and hypoxia.

Intraoperatively a tension pneumothorax may occur in patients with a simple pneumothorax who are ventilated, or who receive nitrous oxide. Tension pneumothorax is a cause of shock. If the air is under pressure the lung will collapse and mediastinal shift and venous obstruction may cause cardiovascular collapse.

Diagnosis
The differential diagnosis includes other causes of shock, airway obstruction, and accidental bronchial intubation.

A reduction in breath sounds, hyperresonant percussion note, and difficulty in ventilating may indicate development of pneumothorax. Simple pneumothorax may require chest X-ray to confirm the diagnosis.

Tension pneumothorax is a clinical diagnosis: progressively increasing airway pressures, hypoxia, hypotension and mediastinal shift.

Treatment
Give 100% oxygen, stop nitrous oxide.

The emergency treatment of a tension pneumothorax is decompression by needle thoracentesis: a 14-gauge cannula connected to a 10 ml syringe is inserted in the 2nd intercostal space in the mid-clavicular line. The gas under tension is allowed to come out via the cannula (the patient will now have a 'simple' pneumothorax).

A simple pneumothorax is treated by insertion of a chest drain usually through the 5th intercostal space in the mid-axillary line, and connected to an underwater seal.

A chest X-ray is performed afterwards to confirm correct placement of the drain and resolution of the pneumothorax.

27. POSTOPERATIVE NAUSEA AND VOMITING (PONV)

Definition
Nausea or vomiting in the postoperative period.

Clinical features
Certain patients are more at risk: females, pregnancy, history of motion sickness or previous PONV, diabetes, obesity, and non-smokers.
Some procedures predispose to PONV: laparoscopic surgery, strabismus surgery, orchidopexy, middle ear surgery and lithotripsy.
Some anaesthetic techniques increase the risk: opioids, nitrous oxide, etomidate, ketamine and neostigmine.
Postoperative factors: pain, sudden movement, hypotension, hypoxia, hypoglycaemia, gastric distension and swallowed blood in the stomach.

Diagnosis
The diagnosis is usally clear-cut. It is important to exclude a surgical cause such as intestinal obstruction.

Action
Reversible causes (gastric distension, hypovolaemia, hypoglycaemia, pain) should be treated before administering antiemetics.
It is better to prevent PONV, and in established PONV it is better to use a different antiemetic if one has failed to be effective. High-risk cases (with two or more of the above risk factors) should be given prophylactic antiemetics before the end of the procedure.
The following antiemetics are used (your hospital may have its own protocol):

- Cyclizine 50 mg i.v.; can be repeated every 6–8 h; particularly effective against PONV associated with use of opioid drugs. Side-effects include tachycardia, dry mouth, extrapyramidal effects and drowsiness.
- Selective 5-HT$_3$ receptor antagonists: granisetron 1 mg i.v. effective for up to 18 h, and often used for prophylaxis; ondansetron 4 mg i.v. effective for 4–6 h. These agents lack the sedative, dysphoric and extrapyramidal effects of other antiemetics, therefore can be used in combination with cyclizine in resistant cases.
- Haloperidol 1.25 mg i.v.; may cause sedation.
- Metoclopramide 10–20 mg i.v.; not as effective as drugs above.
- Dexamethasone 4 mg i.v.; used as a rescue medication for intractable cases.

In general, use of combination therapy is more efficacious than single therapy. Many of the above drugs can be repeated if the first dose has no or little effect.

28. PROLONGED SURGERY

Definition
No simple definition.

Clinical features

Temperature
Risk of hypothermia (core temperature <35°C) which may lead to decreased drug metabolism (e.g. non-depolarizing relaxants), excess oxygen requirements and myocardial work during rewarming, reduced blood flow, abnormalities of haemostasis.
Anaesthesia inhibits normal thermoregulation.
Higher risk if open body cavity, neonates, burns patients.

Pressure area care
These can be on any dependent part, e.g. sacrum, heels, occiput, and areas resting against hard objects, e.g. elbows.

Accumulation of drugs
Many drugs will accumulate, particularly those which are fat-soluble such as volatile agents.
Others display prolonged elimination with increasing doses, e.g. opioids.
The result is a prolonged recovery, and persistent drowsiness.

Action

Temperature
Space blankets, warming blankets, forced warm air devices, wrapping the head etc., heating fluids, and a heat and moisture exchanger in the airway help maintain temperature. The temperature should be monitored in long duration operations.

Pressure areas
Prevention includes use of adequate padding, careful positioning and ripple mattresses.

29. PULMONARY EMBOLISM

Definition
Pulmonary embolism can result from thrombus, fat (see section on orthopaedic surgery), air (see air embolism) or amniotic fluid. The common use of the term usually refers to embolus of a thrombus.

Clinical features
The usual sources of thromboemboli are deep venous thrombosis in the legs, pelvis or lower extremities.

Factors which promote thrombus formation are: stasis of blood, hypercoagulable state, fracture of the lower limbs or pelvis, pregnancy, malignancy and the oral contraceptive.

Significant pulmonary embolus causes ventilation/perfusion mismatch and hypoxia, tachypnoea and tachycardia.

The ECG may show right axis deviation, right bundle branch block and anterior T wave changes.

Diagnosis
Unexplained hypoxia.

A sudden reduction in end-tidal carbon dioxide (due to an increase in dead-space).

Signs of deep vein thrombosis.

Pulmonary angiography.

Management
Mainly supportive.

100% oxygen.

Intravenous fluids and inotropes.

For severe hypoxia or cardiovascular collapse consider embolectomy or extracorporeal oxygenation.

Systemic heparinization or thrombolysis may not be an option in patients undergoing surgery.

30. SUXAMETHONIUM APNOEA

Definition
Muscle relaxation of longer duration than planned due to an inherited (autosomal recessive) abnormality of suxamethonium metabolism.

Clinical features
Muscle relaxation after a standard dose of suxamethonium that lasts longer than the usual 5–10 min.

The prolongation may be minutes or hours depending on the exact genotype. There are a number of abnormal genes known.

The normal genotype is present in about 94% of the population. Heterozygotes for the commonest abnormal gene (approximately 4% of the population) have apnoea after suxamethonium for 10–30 min.

The rarer genotypes may lead to apnoea lasting several hours.

Plasma cholinesterase deficiency may also be acquired with:

- liver failure
- renal disease
- malnutrition
- pregnancy
- hypothyroidism
- use of anticholinesterases and organophosphorus drugs, e.g. ecothiopate.

Diagnosis
Prolonged muscle paralysis diagnosed by bedside evaluation of neuromuscular function.

Confirmed by plasma cholinesterase assay to determine genotype.

May be determined preoperatively in at-risk individuals (i.e. family members of index cases).

Action
Make correct diagnosis.

Ensure adequate ventilation.

Ensure adequate anaesthesia/sedation to prevent awareness.

Take blood for plasma cholinesterase assay.

Fresh frozen plasma may be used to reverse block if necessary – but the risk of a transfusion must be considered against what is a self-limiting condition that should not be associated with any morbidity or mortality.

Screen near relatives.

31. TRANSFUSION REACTIONS

Definition
A reaction due to transfusion of blood or blood products. Can be haemolytic, allergic or febrile.

Clinical features
Haemolytic transfusion reactions result from transfusion of serologically incompatible blood and can lead to haemolysis of donor erythrocytes. The mortality rate is 20–60%.

Can present as fever, hypotension, tachycardia, unexplained bleeding, and haemoglobinuria (urine may be red or brown black).

One of the commonest causes remains administrative failure leading to transfusion of incompatible blood.

Allergic transfusion reaction can arise from various proteins in donor plasma. Transfusion of fresh frozen plasma, packed RBCs and platelets can all cause allergic reactions.

Manifestations range from mild reactions such as flushing, rash and urticaria to severe cases with bronchospasm, laryngeal oedema and anaphylactic shock.

Febrile transfusion reactions are usually due to leucocyte containing/contaminated blood products producing an antigen-antibody reaction characterized by a temperature increase of >1°C.

Febrile reactions are usually benign; hypotension is rare and treatment is with an antipyretic.

Diagnosis
Depends on a high index of suspicion during any transfusion of blood products.

For suspected haemolytic and allergic reactions blood and urine samples should be sent for evidence of haemolysis (plasma and urine haemoglobin, haptoglobin, bilirubin).

Unused donor blood along with a fresh blood sample from the patient should be sent for re-cross matching.

Empty bags of all blood products along with labels should be sent for examination.

Action
Stop transfusion.

Administer oxygen.

Use fluids and vasopressors to treat hypotension.

Maintain urine output with diuretics and mannitol.

Consult haematologist and intensivists – renal support or even exchange transfusion may be required.

Monitor and treat coagulation problems.
Monitor and treat renal function.
Treat severe allergic reactions with epinephrine, fluids, steroids and antihistamines (similar to management of anaphylactic shock).

32. VOMITING AND REGURGITATION

Definition

Regurgitation is the passive movement of stomach contents up the oesophagus under hydrostatic pressure into the mouth and pharynx.

Vomiting is the active propulsion of stomach contents up the oesophagus (it does not occur in the fully anaesthetized state).

Aspiration is the entrance of food or liquid into the trachea and lower airways.

Clinical features

Vomiting is an active process in the awake or partially anaesthetized patient. Regurgitation is often silent and only detected when the mouth is opened and examined. Clinical features of aspiration include bronchospasm, hypoxia, tachypnoea, atelectasis, tachycardia and hypotension.

Patients at increased risk of aspiration include pregnant women, the obese, history of recent ingestion of food, hiatus hernia or intestinal obstruction.

The clinical course depends upon the volume and pH of the aspirated material.

Diagnosis

Diagnosis of significant aspiration can be difficult and may be made retrospectively.

Suctioning of obvious food residues or an acidic fluid from the trachea.

Action

Vomiting and regurgitation

Place the patient into the Trendelenburg (head-down) position to minimize passive flow of gastric contents into the trachea.

Turn the head to one side, or roll the patient into the left lateral position.

If not intubated, apply cricoid pressure and secure the airway by tracheal intubation.

Gently suction the lower airway before commencing positive pressure ventilation.

Aspiration

100% inspired oxygen.

Bronchodilators.

Frequent suctioning of the airway.

Chest X-ray for evidence of collapse of lung segments.

Bronchoscopy and toilet, especially if gastric contents contained particulate material.

The use of prophylactic antibiotics is controversial – take advice from local microbiologist.

Consider the use of steroids (unproven benefit).

Arrange intensive observation and care in ICU or HDU.

(Late complications such as pneumonia, ARDS, secondary organ failure requiring inotropes are associated with a high mortality.)

INDEX

Unanticipated difficult tracheal intubation–during rapid sequence induction of anaesthesia in non–obstetric adult patient

```
Direct          →    Any          →    Call
laryngoscopy          problems          for help
```

Plan A: Initial tracheal intubation plan

Pre-oxygenate
Cricoid force: 10N awake → 30N anaesthetised
Direct laryngoscopy – check:
Neck flexion and head extension
Laryngoscopy technique and vector
External laryngeal manipulation –
by laryngoscopist
Vocal cords open and immobile
If poor view:
Reduce cricoid force
Introducer (bougie) – seek clicks or
hold-up and/or Alternative
laryngoscope

Not more than
3 attempts,
maintaining:
(1) oxygenation
with face mask
(2) cricoid
pressure and
(3) anaesthesia

— Succeed → Tracheal intubation

Verify tracheal intubation
(1) Visual, if possible
(2) Capnograph
(3) Oesophageal detector
"If in doubt, take it out"

Plan C: Maintenance of oxygenation, ventilation, postponement of surgery and awakening

Failed intubation

Maintain 30N cricoid force

Plan B: not appropriate for this scenario

Use face mask, oxygenate and ventilate
1 or 2 person mask technique
(with oral ± nasal airway)
Consider reducing cricoid force
if ventilation difficult

— Succeed →

Failed oxygenation
(e.g. SpO_2 < 90% with FiO_2 1.0)
via face mask

LMA™
Reduce cricoid force during insertion
Oxygenate and ventilate

— Succeed →

Failed ventilation and oxygenation

Plan D: Rescue techniques for can't intubate, can't ventilate situation

Postpone surgery
and awaken patient if possible
or continue anaesthesia with
LMA™ or ProSeal LMA™ –
if condition immediately
life-threatening